THE NEW RULES OF RUNNING

THE NEW RULES OF RUNNING

Five Steps to Run Faster and Longer for Life

VIJAY VAD, MD

with Dave Allen

AVERY
a member of Penguin Group (USA)
New York

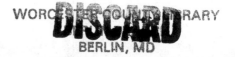

Published by the Penguin Group
Penguin Group (USA) LLC
375 Hudson Street
New York, New York 10014

USA • Canada • UK • Ireland • Australia
New Zealand • India • South Africa • China

penguin.com
A Penguin Random House Company

Most Avery books are available at special quantity discounts for bulk purchase for sales promotions, premiums,
fund-raising, and educational needs. Special books or book excerpts also can be created to fit specific needs.
For details, write Special.Markets@us.penguingroup.com

Library of Congress Cataloging-in-Publication Data

Vad, Vijay.
The new rules of running : five steps to run faster and longer for life / Vijay Vad, Dave Allen.
p.   cm.
ISBN 978-1-58333-538-3 (pbk.)
1. Running—Physiological aspects.   2. Running injuries—Prevention.   3. Running injuries—Treatment.   4. Running—
Handbooks, manuals, etc.   5. Runners (Sports)—Handbooks, manuals, etc.   I. Allen, Dave,   II. Title.
RC1220.R8V34   2014   2013043693
617.1'027—dc23

Printed in the United States of America
1   3   5   7   9   10   8   6   4   2

BOOK DESIGN BY TANYA MAIBORODA

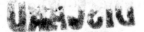

I dedicate this book to my children,

Amoli and Nikhil,

who have inspired me to run like a child again.

May they continue the tradition of running as a family.

Contents

THE NEW RULES OF RUNNING

Introduction

Running: The Ultimate Mind-Body Tune-Up

PEOPLE HAVE MANY DIFFERENT REASONS FOR RUNNING. THEY RUN TO stay healthy and in shape, or to lose weight, or to scratch that competitive itch they might be having. Others run because it's a good way to relieve stress—to decompress from the pressures of their everyday lives. Still others run for social reasons—to spend time with friends—or because it simply makes them feel good about themselves.

I run because it's the ultimate fitness activity. It's one of the best core exercises you can do, and it really gets the blood pumping through your body, which is good for your heart and your lungs. Running, along with other intensive sports activities like cross-country skiing, interval training, biking, and mountain climbing, is known to increase your maximum aerobic capacity, or VO_2 max levels, which is a measurement of your lungs' ability to use oxygen.

I also run because it's a great way to spend quality family time with my two young children. Every Saturday (except in the cold winter months), we head to Central Park and run the reservoir loop—a 1.58-mile track with breathtaking views of the park and New York City skyscrapers. My son, Nikhil, who is 6, can run a 10-minute mile now without breaking a sweat. And my daughter, Amoli, who is 7, can't wait to put on her shoes and head out the door. She craves running. Not only does she look like an athlete now, but she also has a focus and discipline that are so much better today than they were several years ago. It used to be that she'd get bored and move on to something else fairly quickly, but now, because of the running, she can focus on an individual task for several hours. And she really enjoys it. She said as much to me recently, telling me, "Dad, I like running because it is fun and is good for you." My original hope was that if I got them to run at such a young age, they'd develop a passion for a healthy activity they could enjoy for a lifetime. But I never thought it would have the impact it's had.

Last, I run because it's convenient and fairly inexpensive. I don't need a partner or a teammate, nor do I have to join a gym or pay an admission fee to go run in one of the world's most stimulating settings, Central Park. I simply lace up my running shoes, jog a few blocks over to the park's main drive or reservoir, and run.

Chances are that if you're reading this book, you, too, are running for one or more of the aforementioned reasons. Well, I'm about to give you a few more reasons why you should continue to run—not just now but also in the many years to come. It has recently come to light that running, in addition to increasing endurance and leading to better overall physical conditioning, can have a similarly positive impact on the brain. There's growing evidence that running and other forms of exercise can improve your cognitive functioning and lower your risk of developing Alzheimer's disease and other mental illnesses often associated with aging. It can combat depression and make you smarter and more focused—as shown by my daughter's experience.

One recent study conducted by Nihon Fukushi University in Japan shows the impact that moderate, sustained running can have on your brain. Seven young adults were asked to embark on a 3-month jogging program in which they would run for 30 minutes two to three times per week. The participants were given a computer-based series of tests before and after the jogging program, and their test scores improved substantially with running. Once they stopped training, however, their performance began to decline. In other words, running improved their cognitive functioning (i.e., memory and focus), but only if they maintained some form of conditioning.

In another recent study, researchers discovered that laboratory mice that were bred to run had a 13 percent larger midbrain than normal, untrained mice. Besides controlling your body's visual and auditory systems, the midbrain also releases a chemical, or neurotransmitter, called dopamine, which sends signals to other nerve cells that the body interprets as a reward. In other words, it's very similar to adrenaline.

Running has similarly been shown to increase the production of endorphins, another neurotransmitter secreted within the brain and nervous system that helps block pain and produce a feeling of well-being. This is where the term "runner's high" comes from: The brain releases these endorphins to give you the high—a very pleasurable, orgasmic post-run feeling. It is also why many scientists believe that running is a very effective way to curb depression.

So there you have it; the evidence is overwhelming: Running is not only a great way to exercise but also one of the best forms of mind-body therapies there is. Now that you know just how wonderful this sport is for you, it's time to see if we can get you running faster and more efficiently than ever before. Because when it comes down to it, most runners are on a high the minute they participate in their first road race. They're instantly hooked for life, and they want to know how they can run their next race faster, and run longer.

The New Rules of Running provides strategies to get the very best performance out of your body, with exercises to boost your VO_2 max level—your fuel tank—and strengthen those all-important core muscles, which are prone to fatigue. It also includes essential nutrition and hydration tips to fuel and nourish your body so that you don't wind up cramping, hitting the wall, or getting injured. For middle- and long-distance runners, we have full training schedules for the half-marathon and full marathon, with the focus on maximizing peak performance and preventing injuries. There's also a low-mileage training plan for those people looking to use running as a way to lose weight or sustain a healthy level of fitness.

Now, let's get you started.

1

The Five New Rules
of Running

THE NUMBER OF AMERICANS RUNNING MARATHONS HAS INCREASED BY almost a half million in the past 35 years, from as few as 25,000 in 1976 to 518,000 in 2011. One of the reasons for the growing popularity of this 26.2-mile race and the even more popular 13.1-mile half-marathon is middle-age Americans' increased fascination with endurance sports. More and more baby boomers and Generation X men and women are competing in marathons, triathlons, and Ironmans than ever before, and the average age of the first-time marathoner is creeping upward, with some crossing the finish line for the first time in their 40s and 50s.

Of the nearly half-million Americans who completed a marathon in 2012, about half (46 percent) were over the age of 40. In fact, the second-largest group of finishers in the 2012 Chicago Marathon were males ages 40 to 49; they trailed only males ages 30 to 39. The average median age of the marathoner in 2012 was 38.3 years, 39.8 years for men and 36.2 for women.

Why the interest in endurance sports later in life? First, there's a desire to be fit and healthy, as we were in our younger years. But another contributing factor is that as we get older, we have more disposable income and time. Those in their 20s and 30s have much less of both; they're fighting to establish a career and earn a living, while in many instances raising children. The latter may explain the explosive growth of female long-distance runners in the past two decades. In 2011, the number of women who finished road races was an all-time high of 7,685,700, or 55 percent of all finishers. In 1990, women represented as little as 25 percent of finishers. What's more, women composed 59 percent of the more than 1.6 million people who finished half-marathons in 2011, up from 49 percent in 2004. As children get older and become more capable of taking care of themselves, parents have more time to devote to improving their own overall fitness, and many find running the fastest and most convenient way to do so.

The relative simplicity of distance running is a lure for many adults, who see it as a second sporting life, if you will. Road racing is a way of scratching a competitive itch that might still be burning, especially when the other sports you played growing up (soccer, basketball, football, etc.) become too inconvenient and hard on your body. Running a 5K or 10K is manageable, and so, too, apparently, is finishing a marathon. Outside of the Ironman, the marathon is the ultimate test of endurance, yet the numbers continue to suggest that you don't have to be in your 20s to run 42 kilometers. Would you believe that almost 2,500 runners over the age of 60 completed the 2011 Honolulu Marathon?

It's no coincidence, however, that as the age of people running distance races has increased, so, too, have the median finish times. In 1995, it took men an average of 3:54:00 to finish a marathon and women an average of 4:15:00; in 2012, those numbers grew to 4:17:43 and 4:42:58, respectively. In many instances, you can attribute these slower times to the democratic process of running a marathon and the sheer size of fields today. As many as 16 marathons had more than 15,000 finishers in 2011. And no one is prohibited from walking a marathon, which many entrants in the larger marathons do. Yet there's no arguing with the fact that age does affect performance, and more specifically, endurance.

As you get older, your maximum heart rate begins to decline; thus, so does the intensity at which you're able to run and work out. Your hormone levels (testosterone in men, estrogen in women) also begin to fall, which leads to a loss of approximately 1 percent of muscle mass per year starting around the age of 40. Further-more, your tissues—especially your cartilage, tendons, and ligaments—begin to lose water content (about 1 percent per year), and the blood flow to your tendons also diminishes. Add it all up, and you can see why you have such a hard time recovering from your workouts and why you're more prone to injury later on in life.

But just because you're older doesn't mean you can't run faster or more efficiently than ever before. There are thousands of stories of runners who established new personal bests in their 40s and 50s and who are running faster and longer than they did when they were much younger. Some of the world's best long-distance runners didn't find the fountain of youth until they hit their 30s. American Deena Kastor was 31 when she won a bronze medal in the marathon at the 2004 Summer Olympic Games in Athens, and two years later she set an American record in the London Marathon. Fellow American Meb Keflezighi won the 2009 New York City Marathon at 34, and in 2012, at age 36, became the oldest winner of the Olympic marathon trials, held in Houston, when he established a new personal best of 2:09:08. Several months later, he placed fourth in the London Olympic Games.

No matter what age you begin to run, or what reason you have for running, you can become better at it. That's why you picked up this book. You have a certain goal you'd like to achieve, whether it is completing your first marathon or half-marathon, setting a new personal record in your next 10K, or simply avoiding those injuries that always seem to dog you in training. It might be that you want to improve your overall fitness or learn how to run more frequently so that you can lose weight. Perhaps you've run one or more races in the past and you're looking for ways to get you to the finish line faster and with less pain.

The New Rules of Running will help you to do all of those things and to accomplish whatever goals you've set going forward. It's chock-full of new research on how to train better and run longer and healthier for life.

As you page through this book, you'll often see references to the five rules that follow. Consider these rules your lifeline to running. In other words, anytime you have a question about nutrition or hydration, or you're just not sure how to proceed with your training, turn to these rules for help. They will serve as a mentor of sorts, keeping you on the proper path as you pursue your running goals.

Rule No. 1: There's No One Way to Run

Tom Fleming, a two-time winner of the New York City Marathon and the architect of the training programs you'll see later in this book, has a unique hobby: He likes to watch people walk and run. As a personal coach and the head coach of the varsity cross-country and indoor and outdoor track and field teams at Montclair Kimberley Academy in New Jersey, it's his job to observe his runners in action and to offer guidance on how to best improve their form and efficiency. And sometimes he just can't leave his job at the office. One of the world's best marathoners in the 1970s, Fleming says he can tell a lot about people just by the way they walk—how fast their gait is, how they carry their arms, etc. For example, if he sees someone with a quick arm swing, he knows that person will typically have a fast leg motion.

Tom will tell you that he can see these patterns in someone as early as age 2, and he's right. By the time you're 15 months old, you've already developed a fairly consistent walk, or gait pattern. The "stance and swing" phase of your walking and running cycle is refined as your body begins to grow and develop, but once you're through puberty, you've largely established what type of runner you're going to be. The runner you are today is more a product of nature (i.e., your body type) than it is of nurture. Everything from your arch type to your posture to the alignment of your knees and hips to the length of your legs relative to your torso plays a part in defining you as a runner. That's why if you stand at the finish line of any marathon, you see all different styles of runners.

In an ideal world, you'd have a fast foot turnover and a very long stride, your feet would barely touch the ground, and you'd look effortless in full flight—like the world's fastest man, Usain Bolt. But if you're 6-foot-4 and built like an offensive tackle, you're not going to run like a bolt of lightning; and if you're 5 feet, 100 pounds and built like a world-class gymnast, you're not going to outstride anyone. You have to make do with the body type that you were born with, and make it as efficient as possible.

I can't change the type of runner you are, but I can make your movements more economical by teaching you better posture and mechanics and sharing with you all the latest science on how to increase strength and endurance, and prevent and treat injuries. While there is no one most efficient way to run, there is a most efficient way of running for you, and *The New Rules of Running* will point you in the right direction.

Rule No. 2: Speed Is Strength in Disguise

After Bill Rodgers won the 1975 Boston Marathon with a then-American record time of 2:09:55, he called his time "absurd." "I can't run that fast," said the four-time winner of both the Boston and New York City Marathons. "I must be dreaming this whole thing."

Not far behind Rodgers, in third place, was Tom Fleming, who established a personal-best time of 2:12:05. Of the 2,340 starters in the field that year, 113 finished in under 2 hours, 30 minutes. It was the fastest mass marathon to date, according to the Boston Athletic Association. In 2011, 36 years later, only 92 runners (out of field of nearly 24,000) broke the 2:30 barrier. The times at the top were faster—Kenya's Geoffrey Mutai ran the fastest marathon in history (2:03:02)—but the overall depth of talent wasn't as good as it was when Rodgers crossed the tape in 1975. In the 2012 marathon, in extremely warm temperatures, only 21 runners finished in under 2:30.

"We had more quality runners back then because we did more running," says Fleming, who climbed to as high as number 4 in the world rankings. "We ran farther. Bill and I tried a lot of different things, but we figured we were going to go out and train more than anyone else."

In many ways, this "new" rule is an old rule that took shape in the late 1960s, when several elite distance runners, including Fleming, Rodgers, and Amby Burfoot, started training under a method referred to as long, slow distance (LSD). They believed that by running at a more leisurely pace, approximately 50 to 60 seconds slower than their own marathon pace, they would have the ability to dramatically increase their weekly mileage. Did they ever! Fleming and Rodgers once logged a staggering 210 miles in one week, running 30 miles per day. (They would break it up into either three 10-mile runs or two 15-milers.) That distance proved to be too much, and eventually they trimmed it down to about 160 miles per week—slightly more than what most elite marathoners run today.

Of the 160 miles Fleming ran each week, very few were at or faster than his marathon race pace (5 minutes per mile). He would run a few 4:40 to 4:50 pickups mid-run, but for the most part, his training runs averaged 5:50 to 6 minutes per mile. Fleming believed—as did Rodgers and Burfoot, Rodgers's teammate at Wesleyan University in Connecticut—that speed is strength in disguise, and that by running at a pace that can be easily sustained over a longer haul, you can improve your aerobic fitness and your ability to run faster and more efficiently. Burfoot had trained under the LSD method when he captured the Boston Marathon in 1967.

"I ran my personal-best mile of 4:09:02 when I was training long, slow distance for a marathon," Fleming says. "I never saw the other side of 6 minutes [per mile] when I was training, but that was well within my comfort zone. Some days when you're training and you're tired, 6 miles at any pace is hard."

Fleming firmly believes that if you have a good, strong base, you can run your personal best for a marathon, a 10K, a 5K, or even a mile, as he did. "Fitter equals faster," he says. "The speed will come from running lots of miles."

Fleming doesn't suggest that you run 160 miles per week, like he once did. "Everyone is different and has to find their own ceiling," he says. But running the vast majority of your miles at race pace or faster and incorporating too much speed-work into your program are how the average runner finds him- or herself in the doctor's office instead of on the course come race day. Too many intermediate and first-time marathoners run their training miles at marathon pace or faster. They are coached by their GPS watches, says Fleming, and they often get injured as a result.

Now, you can't just run and do nothing else: You also need to supplement your mileage with a program that emphasizes strength and resistance training (i.e., eccentric contractions, in which the muscle is actively lengthening; also known as the "negative" phase). Typically, the first muscles to fatigue when you run are the hip abductors, and the more endurance you build in these, the longer you'll be able to maintain your posture and center of gravity, and the more efficiently you will run. Other core muscles, like your hip flexors and gluteus maximus, also need to be trained so that you can maintain your knee lift and proper leg stride as you run longer distances. (For more on these training exercises, see chapter 5.)

Rule No. 3: You Must Learn to Endure

Ever wonder why the Kenyans dominate the middle-distance and long-distance events worldwide, and not the equally talented runners from Ecuador, Chile, Mexico, and other high-altitude countries? It's because the Kenyans run more than anyone else, and they start at a younger age. As a result, their engines are bigger and faster than everyone else's, meaning their VO_2 max levels—the measure of your lung capacity and how much oxygen your body is able to utilize—are superior to those of runners from most other countries. As Fleming says, "Would you rather go into battle with a tank or a jeep?" The Kenyans have the former.

By definition, endurance is the ability to repeat an activity over and over again for a long period of time, and to do that, you need a well-tuned cardiopulmonary system along with a strong, supporting musculoskeletal system. The higher your VO_2 max levels, the more energy you'll be able to produce and the longer you'll be able to endure during high-intensity exercise, such as running a 5K or 10K or a marathon.

Fleming equates endurance with what he calls "on-your-feet time." If you were to stand on your feet for 4 hours, you would become very fatigued just by the effects of gravity pulling you down. Now imagine running on your feet for 4-plus hours! Remember from earlier, the average finishing time for a marathon in 2012 was 4:17:43 for men and 4:42:58 for women. If you want to be among these finishers or you want to improve on your previous time, then you have to prepare your body to be on your feet for 3, 4, 5, or however many hours you think it will take you to complete the marathon.

By gradually increasing the amount of on-your-feet running time—say, first to 90 minutes, then to 2 hours, then to 2:10, 2:20, and so on—you can get someone who's never run a marathon acclimated to being on their feet for as many as 3 hours. Training for any longer than 3 hours is senseless and leaves you more susceptible to injury, Fleming says. So how does a 4-hour-plus marathoner finish if he or she has never run for longer than 3 hours? Adrenaline, for one, Fleming says, but all of those miles logged during several months of training is what will ultimately carry them across the finish line.

Rule No. 4: Hydrating and Eating Properly Stimulate Recovery

Dehydration is a big problem with runners, especially those who train for long-distance races. Fluids are essential to maintaining the contraction and relaxation of your muscles, and when you don't consume enough water and electrolytes, the flow of electrical impulses that powers your muscles and tendons is impaired. This can cause your muscles to cramp and fatigue, and it can lead to strains and other serious running injuries.

You need to be especially cognizant of replenishing electrolytes as you run, because a depletion of magnesium, potassium, and sodium, in particular, can exacerbate these cramps. When you sweat, you lose these valuable electrolytes, which are responsible for transmitting electrical signals within the body; therefore, the more salts and minerals you take in, the less chance you have of cramping. As a general rule of thumb, the warmer it is and the longer you run, the more electrolytes you should consume. Some of the best sports drinks for hydrating and replacing electrolytes on the go include Gatorade, Gatorade Endurance Formula (which has more electrolytes than regular Gatorade), Powerade, and coconut water (a natural source of electrolytes). If none of these liquids is available to you, then you can consume salt tablets or gels that are very high in sodium, such as PowerBar Energy Gel (which has 200 milligrams of sodium).

It's of the utmost importance that our bodies are properly hydrated as we get older, since, besides the risks associated with dehydration, our tissues tend to start losing water after the age of 40. This causes our muscles to become more rigid, like a piece of gum that's been chewed for hours. The fluid within our spinal discs also starts to dry up and become less flexible, making us more susceptible to lower back problems and joint problems as well. It's a process you can't reverse, but it's one you can slow down by staying properly hydrated. On average, you should drink at least ½ ounce of water per day for every pound you weigh in the summer, and ¼ ounce per day in cold weather.

As for your diet, there were indications as early as the 1980s that certain foods could combat inflammation, and that body of evidence continues to grow. The reality is that these foods have been available to us for many thousands of years. They are the foods our ancestors ate—fruits, vegetables, and fish, which are natural sources of proteins, carbohydrates, and good fats that promote healing and sustained health.

Unfortunately, the modern American diet consists of too many readily available processed foods that lack the essential vitamins and nutrients that our bodies need to energize our runs and also to recover from them. In fact, many of the foods we eat today cause our body's natural defense system to respond in much the same way as it would to a wound or a life-threatening situation. In other words, they aid in the inflammation process; they don't slow it down. Some of these pro-inflammatory foods include meats high in saturated fats, fried foods and other foods cooked in vegetable oils, and foods rich in trans fat (an unsaturated fat that is known to raise levels of "bad" low-density-lipoprotein, or LDL, cholesterol) and high-fructose corn syrup (a sugar sweetener found in soft drinks, cereals, baked goods, and processed foods). The latter is a major reason for our country's growing obesity problem—one in every three Americans is obese, and two in three are overweight.

Outside of rest, one of the best ways to recover from a long run or a hard workout is to eliminate these bad foods and to eat an anti-inflammatory diet full of fresh fruits (berries, apples, oranges, bananas), vegetables (dark-green leafy vegetables like spinach, broccoli, cauliflower), and omega-3 essential fatty acids (cold-water fish like salmon and tuna, flaxseed, walnuts). Studies have shown that people who eat a lot of fish rich in omega-3s are less likely to develop arthritis later in life. Fish and these nutrient-rich fruits and vegetables help fight inflammation, so that the lower back pain you're feeling early on in training doesn't materialize into something bigger that knocks you out of your race altogether.

Rule No. 5: Rest Is Essential for Recovery and Improved Performance

In the introduction, I spoke of all the physiological and mental benefits of running. Among other things, it can make you happier, curb depression, improve your memory and focus, and boost your aerobic performance. It has even been shown to lower your risk of developing Alzheimer's disease and other mental illnesses. But there's a point of diminishing return, and, as with any other recreational activity, if you overdo it and put your body under too much stress too often, running can cause you more harm than good.

The human body is an incredible machine. We tear it down, and then it repairs and rebuilds itself. It constantly adapts to stress, and if we continually stress it in the right way—allowing for an adequate amount of rest and recovery—it rewards us by making our muscles and connective tissues even stronger, so our performance gets stronger. This explains why it's so much easier to run 10 miles after 3 months of training than it is after 4 weeks, and why your 10K times continually get faster with each race.

Russian sports scientist N. Yakovlev's model of training and adaptation underscores the importance of recovery, especially after a hard workout. It basically states that if you present the body with an appropriate amount of stress and then allow an adequate time for recovery, your fitness level will surpass what it was during your prior workout. This is the adaptation taking place. Train too hard for your current level of conditioning and recovery rate, however, and your body is likely to become fatigued and break down.

"A runner is overtraining when they cannot repair their body adequately between bouts of exercise," says Dr. Shawn Williams, PhD, a functional medicine clinician and health science professor at York College of the City University of New York. "This leads to more injuries and often slower healing times due to a weakened parasympathetic [nervous system] response. Since running for long distances causes a lot of micro-trauma, it's imperative to allow adequate healing to take place before the next run."

Healing occurs during rest, or what I like to call "restorative sleep." During this time, the body repairs micro-trauma to the soft tissue (muscles and tendons) caused by running. This process helps prevent delayed-onset muscle soreness (DOMS). While at rest, your body is also rehydrating and working to replenish your energy (glycogen stores). A lot goes on during this recovery phase to get your body physiologically tuned and ready for your next run, something that can't happen if you're immediately following up one hard run with another.

Overtraining is the number-one cause of injuries in runners, and it's why we decided to add 3 days to the normal training "week" in our three marathon training plans in chapter 13. By going to a 10-day week, or "phase," as we like to call it, we're able to fit in an extra day of rest and follow up every long run with an off day and an easy recovery day. This hard-easy-easy system is the same one legendary University of Oregon coach Bill Bowerman implemented with his athletes some 40 years ago, and his runners never got injured. It is my hope and expectation that by practicing the basic recovery strategies outlined later in this book, and by following this rule, you will remain injury-free.

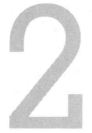

Proper Biomechanics
of Running

WHEN YOU'RE THE WORLD'S FASTEST HUMAN AND A SIX-TIME OLYMPIC gold medalist, every runner looks up to you. And in the case of Usain Bolt, this has never been more true. You see, Bolt, the world record-holder at 100 and 200 meters, is 6-foot-5, 210 pounds, and possesses a body that looks more suited to the football field than the track. Indeed, Bolt would strike a very imposing figure if he lined up as a wide receiver in the National Football League.

Most top distance runners are about 9 or 10 inches shorter than Bolt, and a lot leaner. They don't look like Hercules because it's generally accepted that the thinner you are, the more efficient you'll be over the long haul. But in the short sprinting events, size does matter. Once Bolt gets rolling, the long-limbed Jamaican takes the least amount of steps to go from 0 to 100 meters. He takes 41 steps, whereas the rest of the world's best average about 44. (The runner-up to Bolt in the 2012 100-meter Olympic final, his fellow countryman Yohan Blake, took 46.) Bolt's longer stride, coupled with his tremendous core and upper-body strength, makes him very explosive and economical for the distance he runs.

I bring up the example of Bolt not only because he is unique but also because every runner is different. As renowned running coach Tom Fleming says, "If you stood at the finish line of today's New York City Marathon, you'd see 47,000 different styles of running." Just as each person has a unique set of fingerprints, each person has his or her own individual way of running. No one else on the planet runs exactly the same way you do.

Your running style depends on a number of different things: your physical size and strength, your natural posture, the length of your legs relative to that of your torso, the size of your arch, and the alignment of your knees and hips. For example, Bolt's arms and legs are very long—much longer in proportion to his torso—which explains why he's able to cover ground in fewer steps than all other world-class sprinters. He also has very muscular arms and legs, which is why the 41 steps he does make in the 100 meters are so quick and explosive. He simply rips his cleats off the ground. The faster you swing your arms, the faster your legs are going to move as well.

The single biggest determining factor for what type of runner you'll be is your legs-to-torso ratio—the longer your limbs are, the higher your center of gravity. This not only adds length to your stride but also helps you run faster. Running is a constant up-and-down motion—as you stride forward, your body's mass falls forward, and then it alternatively springs upward. The higher your center of gravity, the faster your body falls forward. Think of yourself jumping into a swimming pool: If you dive into the water off a 3-meter platform, your body is going to be falling forward faster than it would be if you simply dove in off the edge of the pool. It's going to be carrying more forward momentum and thus will generate more speed.

The optimum location for a runner's center of gravity is around the S2 vertebra at the base of the spine, just above the tailbone. A runner with very long legs and a short torso has a higher center of gravity than someone with a larger torso and shorter limbs, even if they're the exact same height. That doesn't mean the long-limbed runner is going to be the faster of the two, however, since there are many other physical and biological factors at play, including age, sex, muscular development, etc. My 7-year-old daughter, Amoli, is all legs and has a small torso; she's a big strider who loves to run. My 6-year-old son, Nikhil, on the other hand, is just the opposite: He has a longer torso and shorter legs, and subsequently has a shorter stride. But he has a perfect arm swing and excellent form when he runs, so he can still motor pretty fast.

While it would be great to go out and precisely mimic Bolt's style, you have a better chance at winning the next half-billion-dollar lottery jackpot. Everybody's running DNA is different. With his longer torso, my son will never make a great sprinter, but that doesn't mean he can't be the fastest kid in his first-grade class. The thing my son and every recreational runner can do is try to emulate certain parts of Bolt's form that will help them become a more efficient runner—i.e., having a high leg kick, a fast arm swing, an upright posture, etc. For each individual, there is a different set of rules, but there is a most efficient way to stride and move your arms, just as there is a most efficient posture and height that you should lift your knees. The purpose of this chapter is to make you aware of these efficiencies so that you can put yourself in position to run your very best. A few subtle changes to your biomechanics may be all you need to achieve your next personal best.

Forefoot vs. Rearfoot Striking

Let's start the discussion on biomechanics from the ground up, since the feet are the only part of your body that actually touch the ground when you're running. Running is different from walking in that it's more of a one-legged exercise—meaning, one leg bears most of your weight every time your foot strikes the ground. Your two feet are never on the ground at the same time. When walking, however, your weight is more evenly distributed over two legs, which alleviates a lot of pressure on your feet and the rest of your body. In a typical walking gait cycle, which begins when one foot strikes the ground and ends when the same foot contacts the ground again, the stance phase (the actual time you're standing on one leg) is approximately 60 percent, whereas the swing cycle, or flight phase (the actual time your leg is swinging forward), is 40 percent. When you are running, however, these numbers tend to be reversed, and the swing cycle is closer to 60 percent.

"The flight phase in running depends on your speed," says Howard Hillstrom, PhD, director of the Leon Root, M.D. Motion Analysis Laboratory at New York City's

Hospital for Special Surgery. "The faster you move, the more time you're in flight and the less time you're in single support [standing on one leg]."

While a person is running, each foot contacts the ground approximately 80 to 100 times per minute on average, according to Peter Larson, author of *Tread Lightly: Form, Footwear, and the Quest for Injury-Free Running*. Put another way, that's 160 to 200 steps per minute, or 9,600 to 12,000 steps per hour of running. Over the course of a 5-hour marathon, that would be approximately 60,000 steps.

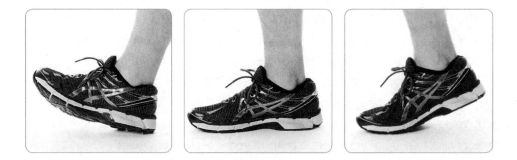

Exactly how your feet strike the ground has a lot to do with what you're wearing on your feet, if anything at all. Wearing modern elevated heel-cushioned shoes, 75 to 80 percent of all runners today are rearfoot strikers, meaning their heel touches down before their forefoot—usually toward the middle or outside of the heel just below the ankle joint. The foot then pronates, or rolls in toward the ankle, bringing the center of pressure in more medially, before toe-off (photo sequence, above). This is generally why you see a diagonal wear pattern across the mid-foot to the big toe on the tread of an older pair of running shoes.

Prior to the invention of the modern running shoe, almost all runners were mid-foot or forefoot strikers, meaning that the heel and ball of their foot land simultaneously or that the ball of their foot lands first. But with an elevated rear sole that's about twice as thick as the sole under the forefoot, today's modern running shoes make it almost impossible not to heel strike.

There is a biomechanical advantage to landing on your forefoot (i.e., a faster toe-off), but recent evidence has come to light showing that forefoot striking can also be safer on your body than rearfoot striking. This would help explain the increasing number of recreational runners switching to barefoot running or minimalist shoes in recent years.

As strange as it might seem to see someone running down the street barefoot, it's hardly anything new. For hundreds of thousands of years, humans ran either barefoot or in minimally soled shoes such as sandals, running flats, or moccasins. To protect their heel, they developed more of a mid- or forefoot strike pattern and made more use of the muscles at the ankle, knee, and hip to absorb shock, Hillstrom says. The human heel alone can't cushion the force of impact like the whole foot can. Once humans started to make paved roads and sidewalks, however, and there was broken glass on the streets to contend with, we started to make heel-cushioned shoes.

The problem with today's modern cushioned running shoes is that while they make the foot strike more comfortable (especially in the heel) and help stabilize the foot, they significantly alter the proper biomechanical workings of the foot, particularly at impact. A lot of the foot-intrinsic muscles are shut off and become atrophied because of the extra cushioning, which ends up putting additional stress on your bones, joints, and tendons. The stronger and more active the muscles in the foot are, the more stable the foot is, and the less likely you are to overpronate.

A study conducted by the Department of Human Evolutionary Biology at Harvard University, titled "Foot Strike Patterns and Collision Forces in Habitually Barefoot versus Shod Runners," concluded that runners who struck the ground consistently with their forefoot were less prone to impact-related injuries of the feet and lower limbs than those who were rearfoot strikers. The primary reason for this is that forefoot strikers have a more plantar flexed foot at impact, meaning the arch of the foot is flat on the ground and the plantar fascia (the thick, fibrous tissue that connects the heel of your foot to the base of your toes) is flexed outward, toward your toes. The plantar fascia is stretched and therefore tensed, which helps the foot bear more of your body's weight and the initial forces applied to your foot and lower leg at impact with the ground. The heel comes down under the control of your calf muscles and Achilles tendon, and then the ankle flexes.

When the heel touches down first, the ankle is dorsiflexed—meaning your heel is moving toward the ground and your toes are pointing upward—and the plantar fascia is in a slightly weaker, shortened state, as is the arch of your foot. As a result, the vertical forces created by impact with the ground are not spread around the foot and lower leg as much as they are in the forefoot strike, which puts more stress on your skeletal system and your body, especially as you run longer. The Harvard study compared the vertical transient force created by the heel strike to that of someone hitting your heel with a hammer using 1.5 to 3 times your own body weight. Comparatively, in the forefoot strike, these impact-forces are as much as 7 times lower, even on hard surfaces, which is akin to someone hitting your heel lightly with a plastic toy hammer.

After reading this, you might be inclined to shed your favorite pair of running shoes and go barefoot, but don't rush into it. The transition to a barefoot or minimalist style of running can take several weeks or months, since you need to gradually build up the strength and endurance of the foot muscles that have been atrophied by years of rearfoot striking. I would recommend walking barefoot (or in minimalist shoes) along the beach or on a track or other non-concrete surface for at least a month before adopting this method, and only then would I start a light running program. I see a lot of injuries—stress fractures, Achilles tendinitis, metatarsalgia (intense pain in the ball of the foot)—to older barefoot or minimalist runners because they simply don't have the bone density or foot structure to support this style of running. If you suffer from osteoporosis, arthritis, or other joint-related issues of the foot, I suggest you stick with the modern heel-cushioned shoe, as it provides better support and shock absorption.

Light on Your Feet

As much discussion as there is today on what part of the foot should strike the ground first, there's little debate as to where it should strike relative to your body. Each foot should make landfall just slightly ahead of your hips (photo, opposite page).

AS YOUR WEIGHT settles over each foot (i.e., mid-stance), the hip on your standing leg should be directly on top of the foot and your shoulders directly over your hips (photo, page 24).

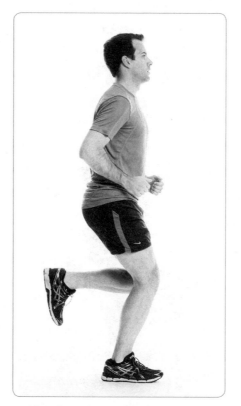

Your foot should strike the ground
slightly ahead of your hips.

YOUR FEET SHOULD land as softly as possible when they touch the ground; they shouldn't make a loud *thud*. The best distance runners in the world are "stealth," Tom Fleming says. They're so light on their feet and their strides are so effortless that when they blow by you, all you feel is the wind. This is why Fleming spends almost as much time listening to his runners as he does watching them.

"In my best races, it seemed like my feet weren't striking the ground real hard," Fleming remembers. "It was like my feet were floating on top of the ground. It was amazing how soft my feet were and how quickly I came up off my toe onto the next step."

"Some people are very heavy and loud when they run," he continues. "You can

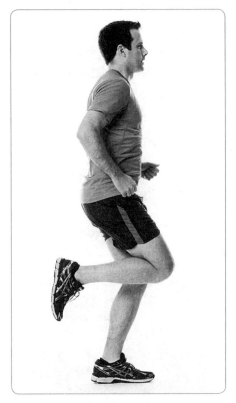

Your upper body should be fairly erect,
with your shoulders over your hips.

hear them coming behind you. And some people you never hear. The people I don't hear are almost always going faster."

Fleming recommends leaving your iPod or MP3 player at home on occasion and listening to the sound of your feet hitting the ground instead. You should try to strike the ground as lightly as you possibly can, maintaining the same gentle "*tit tat tit tat*" sound throughout the entire workout. If you can make sweet music with your feet consistently throughout the run, you should be able to run at a faster, more relaxed tempo (i.e., more efficiently).

Your knees play a vital role in terms of running efficiency as well. As you stride forward, the knee on your swinging leg should come up toward your waist so that the thigh is approximately 45 degrees to the ground (photo, opposite page).

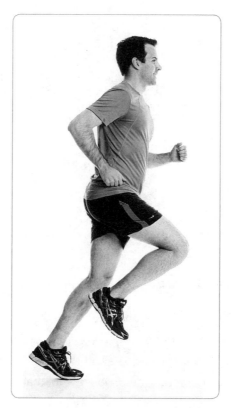

Your swinging leg should form about a
45-degree angle with the ground.

It is this lifting of the knees that propels you forward. One of the biggest signs of fatigue is a low height of the knees—if the knee on your stride leg is barely lifting off the ground, you become more of a shuffler than a runner, and much less efficient. If you want to go faster, you have to lift your knees.

Upper Body: Carry Those Arms

As you run, focus on keeping your upper body over the top of your hips. There should be an ever-so-slight forward lean to your upper body, and your head and chin should be straight. Do not look down at the ground as you run, as this will not only negatively affect your posture, leading to fatigue, but also make it more difficult

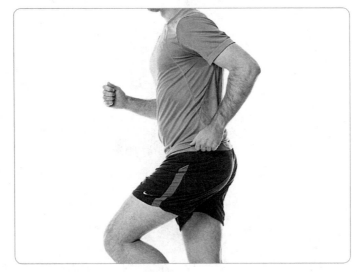

Your palms should face your hips as they pass your waist.

to breathe properly. Fleming recommends looking at a spot on the ground about 10 meters (about 33 feet) ahead of you when you run, which will encourage you to keep your chin up and also allow you to avoid any potential land mines (potholes, rocks, dogs) on the road in front of you. If you're a football fan, think of every down being a first-and-10. Let that imaginary first-down marker, 10 yards in front of you, be your visual reminder to keep your chin up as you run.

How you carry your arms is vital in terms of endurance and speed, and is something you should focus on during your runs, especially when you're getting fatigued. Your arms should be bent 90 degrees at the elbow, but they should be relaxed, not rigid like a robot's. They should swing back and forth in a natural pendulum motion from your shoulders, with very little to no tension. Your hands should be gently balled up into a fist, not clenched, with only your forefingers and thumbs touching very lightly.

VERY IMPORTANT: As your hands pass your waist, your palms should face your hip pockets (photo, above), which helps you to carry your momentum forward and keep your shoulders relatively square. Your hands should finish at mid-chest level

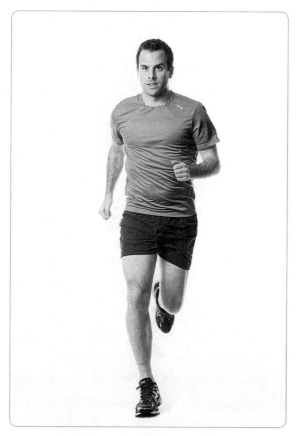

Good form: shoulders square, hands
approach mid-line of chest.

and begin to approach your sternum, but should never cross the midpoint of your chest (photo, opposite page).

If your fists cross the centerline of your body, your shoulders will begin to sway and your body will begin to move sideways, instead of forward. Consequently, you will become less efficient.

You always want to carry your arms forward, so you're directing your body's energy forward.

If you can get your arms moving forward faster, with the palms facing the hip

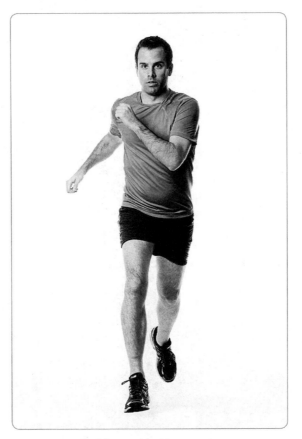

Bad form: shoulders sway,
hands cross mid-line of chest.

pockets, and the fists never crossing the midpoint of your chest, then you will become a faster, more efficient runner. I like to refer to the upper leg muscles and core as the primary engine in a runner, and the arms as the secondary engine. The arms are rocket boosters.

"Your arms dictate what happens below your waist with your legs," Fleming says. "I will rarely say to one of my athletes, 'Move your legs faster.' I will say, 'Move your arms faster.'"

To run faster, Fleming recommends pumping your arms faster—in the efficient manner described above—and taking shorter, quicker strides, not longer ones. The longer the stride, the longer your feet are off the ground and the slower you're going to move. Increase your tempo and the amount of times your feet hit the ground and you'll run faster.

How to Breathe

Going for a run is similar to conducting an orchestra—your arms and legs, as well as your breathing, all need to be in tune with one another if you want to run efficiently. People often ignore the breathing aspect when they're running and, as a result, find themselves extremely tired or gasping for air before their run is over. Your muscles need oxygen to endure, and if they're not getting enough (if, for instance, your breathing is rapid and shallow), they're going to become fatigued sooner.

Your lungs are the primary distributor of oxygen to your heart, your muscles, your brain, and the rest of your body. The greater the intensity of the run, the more oxygen you need to extract from your lungs in order to maintain a sufficient amount of energy. If the effort exceeds the amount of oxygen your muscles are getting, you become fatigued. This is why you might find yourself out of breath when running uphill.

I suggest adopting a 6-second cycle of breathing when running, inhaling through the nose and mouth for a count of 2 seconds, holding that air for 2 seconds, and then exhaling through the nose and mouth for 2 seconds. This will vary somewhat if you're running uphill or at a much slower or faster pace, but the more consistent the pattern, the more efficient you'll be. The reason for holding your breath for 2 seconds is to give your lungs enough time to process the oxygen and allow for an efficient exchange to the blood vessels and then the muscles. If your breathing is rapid and shallow (if you're breathing through your throat or upper chest, not your diaphragm), then your lungs can't dole out enough oxygen to meet the demands placed on your body.

Slippery Slopes

If you've ever run in New York City's Central Park, then you know all about the hills; in particular, the hills at the north end of the park and Cat Hill—a meandering, quarter-mile slope located behind the Metropolitan Museum of Art that often leaves runners gassed and ready to trade in their running shoes for a chairlift. When running any steep incline, you can expect your heart rate and your breathing to increase, so it's important that your cardiovascular system be in tip-top shape. Just as important is your running form: You want to be able to maintain your form so that you can sustain the same pace all the way to the top of the hill. Don't try to lengthen your stride going up the hill; if anything, you want to shorten your stride so that it's easier

THE PERFECT RUNNER'S BODY

A quick glance at the East African male runners dominating the distance events today will tell you that they won't be entering the Mr. Universe bodybuilding contest anytime soon. They all have a similar build, in that they're lean (about 140 to 145 pounds), long-limbed (especially the legs), not particularly muscular, and not very tall (5-foot-8 to 5-foot-9, on average). They're like one of those sleek, new mini-electric cars that get 120 miles per gallon. The top female runners weigh, on average, about 120 to 125 pounds and stand about 5-foot-5 to 5-foot-6.

What makes this type of body ideal for running longer distances? For one, less wear and tear on the body. The impact-forces a lean body endures when each foot strikes the ground are far less than those incurred by a 200-pound individual, making them easier to endure over the course of 10 kilometers, let alone 13.1 or 26.2 miles. Every time your foot strikes the ground, your body is exposed to impact-forces that are 1.5 to 3 times your weight. Since each foot strikes the ground roughly 1,000 times per mile, that's the equivalent of 112.5 to 225 tons of pressure per mile for a 150-pounder, and 150 to 300 tons of pressure for a 200-pounder. The bigger you are, the greater the toll on your body, especially over long distances.

to maintain your tempo. Lean slightly into the hill from your hips, keep your head and chin up, and pump your arms vigorously as you maintain a consistent speed to the top. If you're able to maintain your pace from start to finish, then the hill will go by much faster and you'll also be sure to pick up some time on the rest of the field.

Once you've reached the top of a hill, it's important that you don't relax, so that you can increase your pace simply by allowing the downward momentum of the slope to do its job. Relieved to get the uphill portion done, too many runners "go on vacation" at the hill's apex, says Fleming, and waste valuable time and energy transitioning to the downhill phase. You want to maintain the tempo you established running uphill as you crest the hill and then let gravity kick you into another gear. Again, lean forward so that your body is perpendicular to the hill, and take short, quick strides down the hill—this will happen naturally because your feet will hit the ground faster and more often because of the pull of gravity. Don't consciously try to run faster without maintaining proper form (hips over shoulders, head and chin up, palms facing the hip pockets). Do try to maintain a consistent tempo for the whole duration of the hill.

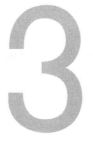

Shoes and Other Running Essentials

WHEN THE GREEK MESSENGER PHEIDIPPIDES RAN FROM THE BATTLE-field in Marathon to Athens in 490 BC to announce the Athenians' victory over the Persians in the Battle of Marathon, he did so barefoot. Legend has it that he ran the entire 40-kilometer (approximately 25-mile) route without stopping, only then to collapse and die after delivering the news.

For thousands and thousands of years, mankind ran barefoot, just as Pheidippides did, or in minimal shoes that offered very little cushioning. Even as late as the 1960 Summer Olympic Games in Rome, gold-medal winner Abebe Bikila of Ethiopia ran the marathon with bare feet. Adidas, the shoe sponsor of those Games, didn't have any shoes that comfortably fit Bikila's feet, so he opted to run in the fashion he had trained in for the race.

Bikila did don a pair of shoes at the 1964 Games in Tokyo, repeating as Olympic champion and setting a new world record in the process. According to the ASICS website, the shoes he wore were manufactured by Onitsuka Tiger, a Japanese shoe outfitter that later merged with two other companies to become the ASICS

Corporation. By the 1976 Summer Games in Montreal, the lightweight shoes with the wafer-thin bottoms, nylon uppers, and tiger stripes (synonymous with ASICS shoes today) were dominating the running shoe market. Coincidentally, the American distributor of the original Onitsuka Tiger running shoe was an Oregon company called Blue Ribbon Sports, which later came to be known as footwear and sportswear apparel giant Nike.

"This was the original running shoe," says multiple-marathon winner Tom Fleming, who ran his first marathon in Tiger stripes. "There was virtually nothing between the ground and my foot, but that's what we all wore back in the late 1960s and early '70s. Today, I can't even walk in those shoes."

Since then, the evolution of the running shoe has come nearly full circle: from an ultra-thin waffle-treaded shoe (Nike cofounder Bill Bowerman found that he could provide better traction by shaping the rubber soles with his wife's waffle iron), to a shoe with a heavily cushioned midsole and heel, to a minimalist shoe with very little support. Today, there's a running shoe for virtually every size and type of runner, from barefoot and trail runners to heavy pronators and road racers. ASICS has eight different categories to fit runner's needs, from Cushioning to Trail to Speed/Lightweight-Minimalist shoes. Brooks and Saucony list as many as eight different types of running shoes, while Nike's website mentions four: Barefoot-like, Stability, Neutral, and Racing.

Due in part to this increased specialization of the running shoe, the industry has become a multibillion-dollar business, with running and jogging shoe sales totaling a record-high $3.04 billion in the United States in 2012, according to the National Sporting Goods Association. That's nearly three times the amount of money that was spent on running and jogging apparel in 2012 ($1.04 billion).

While the clothing you wear to protect yourself from the weather and keep you dry while running is important, it's not as essential. The shoes are the one piece of equipment you're going to use every time you go running—unless you're running barefoot. Therefore, it's the one you want to spend the most time investigating.

The typical runner purchases approximately three pairs of running shoes per year, according to Running USA's 2013 National Runner Survey, and spends roughly $90 plus per pair. So figure that you're going to make an investment of about $300 per year on shoes alone. That's a sizable amount, so you want to take your time in finding a shoe that fits your foot type, is comfortable, and looks good to you.

Which Shoe Is Right for You?

The three basic classifications of running shoes are cushioning, stability, and racing shoes. (Most major shoe manufacturers also sell minimalist and trail shoes.) The first two are training shoes, and that's what the majority of runners wear every day. Most of you who are training for a marathon will be wearing these shoes, too, come race day. These training shoes aren't as cumbersome as they were 10 or 15 years ago. They're relatively lightweight and breathable for all the cushioning and support they provide under the foot, particularly in the midsole. Racing shoes don't have nearly as much cushion in the midsole and are much lighter (most weigh less than 10 ounces) and sleeker in design. They're meant to be worn in competition only, although Fleming believes that it's not worth giving up the extra cushioning and stability of a training shoe unless you plan on running a sub-3-hour marathon.

Minimalist shoes are even lighter—the Nike Free weighs just a little more than 8 ounces—and flex more at the midsole to allow the feet to function in much the same way as if they were bare. These shoes also fit much more snugly to enhance the barefoot-like feel. But as I mentioned in chapter 2, if you are older, have joint issues, or have a tendency to overpronate too much, it's best to stick with a shoe with more support, and always try walking with minimalist shoes on a non-paved surface for at least a month before wearing them on a run.

How do you know which type is right for you? That depends on a number of different factors, including the shape of your arch, your height and weight, and how much running you plan on doing. But, for the most part, your biomechanics dictate what type of shoe you should be in. Most important is how your foot is aligned as it strikes the ground in mid-stance, or when both your heel and toes are on the ground. If your weight is evenly distributed over the foot in mid-stance and the heel slightly pronates, or rolls inward (photos, page 36), then you need a shoe with only a moderate amount of stability—or motion control, as it used to be known.

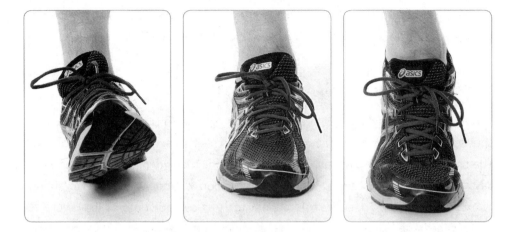

This is typical of runners with a normal-size arch. If, however, your foot over-pronates when it strikes the ground, then you need a shoe with a higher degree of stability. Such shoes have a medial post embedded in the midsole that's firmer than the rest of the midsole or have a firmer midsole under the inner edge of the foot to control the amount of pronation in the arch. People with flat feet tend to be the biggest overpronators.

If you're one of the very few people who supinates, or rolls onto the outside of your arch as you're running, then you need a well-built-up cushioning shoe with very little to no stability. These shoes offer a softer midsole and more flexibility than a stability shoe, so that your foot is able to pronate more naturally. The last thing you want is a rigid pair of shoes that restricts this pronation. Most underpronators have high arches and very rigid ankles. Because their feet do not pronate, they do not absorb shock very well, which is another reason why they need the extra cushioning in the midsole.

If you're not sure what type of arches you have, then take the wet-feet test: Simply lay down a brown paper shopping bag or several pieces of newspaper on the floor just outside your tub or shower, wet the soles of your feet, and stand on the paper. (A thin towel will also work sometimes.) If each foot leaves a half moon–shaped imprint with a thin, elongated heel portion, then you have a normal arch. If the entire underside of the foot makes an imprint, then you have a flat arch. And if only a very narrow portion of the heel and forefoot makes an imprint and the ball of the foot looks like it's detached from the heel, then you have a high arch.

In terms of size, a good rule of thumb is that the heavier you are, the more material, or cushioning, you need between your feet and the ground. If you're 6-foot-2 and weigh 220 pounds, you do not want to be wearing a pair of minimalist or lightweight shoes. You want to be careful, however, not to have too much cushioning, as that tends to immobilize and weaken the feet over time, leaving you more susceptible to injury. In general, a mid-cushion shoe is fine for most runners, although some will need more stability based on their degree of pronation.

Another good rule of thumb is to buy your running shoes at a specialty store, at least until you find a brand and style that is both compatible (i.e., functional) with your feet and comfortable. According to the National Sporting Goods Association, 18 percent of runners purchased their shoes at a specialty athletic footwear store in 2012, down from 19.6 percent in 2011. The advantage to these stores is that they typically have running experts who not only measure your feet but also look at the height of your arches and observe how you walk and run in your shoes. They are able to provide you with the best fit, whereas if you head to the nearest outlet mall to save money, you can't be sure that you'll walk away with the best pair for you.

For many years Fleming owned and operated a specialty running store called Tom Fleming's Running Room in Bloomfield, New Jersey. He sold thousands of shoes, and did so by watching a runner try out a brand-new pair of shoes as well as by carefully examining the runner's current pair—both with their feet in the shoes and out of them. He'd have them walk and run in their old shoes, then he'd remove them to examine the wear patterns on the soles of the shoes. Finally, he'd lay them down flat on the ground to see the degree of either pronation or supination—if the shoe as a whole tilts inward (photo, page 38), the runner pronates, and if it tilts outward, the runner supinates. With all this information, he was then able to recommend certain brands and models.

The lesson here is that you should always bring your current pair of shoes with you if you're thinking of purchasing a new pair of running shoes. Most runners are creatures of habit and will stay with a particular brand and model for as long as

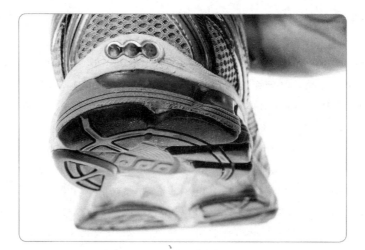

possible, or until the manufacturer alters the line too much. If you find something that gives you enough support and control, that is comfortable, and that looks good to you, then you should stay with it.

The average pair of running shoes today has a life span of approximately 300 to 500 miles, again depending on your size—the larger and heavier you are, the faster the shoe is likely to wear down. If you're in training, make sure to check the soles of your shoes every few weeks for wear and tear. When the outsole of the shoe starts to smooth over like a bald tire, and the ride feels flatter and less cushiony, then it's definitely time to replace your shoes. You should never get to the point where you can see the white midsole layer poking through the outsole. Another good test to see whether it's time for a new pair of shoes is to take the insert out of your shoe and poke your finger around the bottom. If you start to make some kind of indentation in the outsole, then it's clearly time for a change. Your body may also signal when it's time for a new pair. Some typical warning signs that your shoes are getting old include shin splints, sore arches, and aching joints, particularly in the knees.

When you break in a new pair of shoes, Fleming recommends, take the inserts out of your old pair and putting them in your new ones. Since they're already broken in, you'll enjoy a smoother, more comfortable ride while getting the added benefits of a livelier, springier cushioned shoe. Never run a race in a brand-new pair of shoes; you should log at least 50 miles in them beforehand so your feet can get completely acclimated to them.

Other Essential Gear

Just as the number of different types of running shoes has grown rapidly over the past decade, so has the variety of apparel. The materials have become lighter and the colors brighter and more reflective, and there's now a fabric for almost every type of weather condition. High-tech fabrics that keep you cool and dry in the summer and protect you from harsh wind and cold in the winter have replaced cotton, and the days when chafing was as much a part of a long run as "hitting the wall" (a common running term to describe a sudden loss of energy associated with extreme fatigue) are fewer and fewer. Here are a few tips to help you dress for all occasions, from head to toe.

Socks

Stay away from 100 percent cotton and other materials that pick up moisture and cause your feet to sweat. You don't want your socks to bunch up or to slide within the shoe, as that's a surefire way to get a blister. You want moisture-wicking fabrics (Climacool, Coolmax, Dri-FIT, SmartWool, etc.) that pull sweat away from your skin and keep your feet dry. The drier your feet, the less likely there will be any friction between your skin and the material. A number of companies also make right- and left-foot socks, which are specifically designed to fit each foot individually and provide a more secure, comfortable fit.

Shorts/Bottoms

Running capris are very popular with women, since they work well in both winter and summer conditions. These tapered pants are made of stretchy, moisture-wicking fabrics, which help minimize chafing and keep your body cool and dry.

> S teer clear of cotton! Cotton absorbs and holds sweat, causing chafing and adding weight.

Whether shopping for capris or shorts, make sure the seams are flat, since harsh-threaded seams can rub against the skin and irritate it. You also want to make sure there's some kind of cooling effect so that the fabric isn't sticking to your skin, which can also lead to chafing.

Numerous companies, such as CW-X, are building compression into their shorts and leggings. Using body-mapping technology, manufacturers are able to target the parts of the body that are most susceptible to injury, such as the calves, quads, and hamstrings, and to stimulate blood flow to those areas to enhance recovery. The high-compression material hugs the body in these places to increase circulation and range of motion, as well as to provide more support to the muscles and joints and better shock resistance. It works in much the same way as kinesiology therapeutic (KT) athletic tape, which is also popular among runners. If you want even more targeted compression, you can buy compression sleeves for the arms and legs. What's good about these pieces is that they can be easily peeled off and tucked away should you become too hot. For post-run recovery, you can also consider compression stockings, which speed recovery times by stimulating blood flow to the area.

Shirts/Singlets

In the summertime, you want to sport something with minimal coverage. Look for tops that are lightweight, breathable (such as those with mesh fabrics), loose fitting, and of course, sweat wicking. Some fabrics offer additional protection from the sun by having built-in SPF, which is important, especially if you're going to be out there running for 2 or 3 hours. Few people realize that you can get burned through the shirt, especially when you're exposed to the sun for such a long period of time. Stay away from 100 percent cotton and anything that may hug your body too much, especially under the armpits, where it's very easy to chafe. Many companies offer shirts with low-cut armholes, which guard against chafing and are comfortable in hot conditions.

As for running in cold weather, it's essential to keep yourself dry and well insulated, but you don't want to wear too many layers, because you can get very hot, very quickly. Try wearing a moisture-wicking T-shirt under a wool-based zip-up or even a fleece jacket. A lot of today's warmer, sweat-wicking materials are killing the need for three layers.

It's also important to keep your hands, head, and ears well protected. Few things are more painful than cold, wind-burned ears. ASICS makes a pair of mittens that convert to a pair of fingerless gloves so that you can adjust the music on your iPod or MP3 player, something that's difficult to do with normal running gloves. If you prefer not to wear gloves, many long-sleeve tops have a thumbhole built into the cuffs to keep your hands warm.

"These days, no matter the sport, everyone is looking for a combination of looks and comfort," says Argy Koutsothanasis, fashion director at *Fitness* magazine. "Everyone wants to have it be functional and look good. Fortunately, there are so many name brands out there putting out stylish clothes people wear in everyday life that are also performance pieces. The stuff that looks good is the stuff that performs."

GPS Watches/Apps

Outside of your shoes, there's probably nothing more valuable to marathon training than a GPS-enabled watch. These watches do more than tell the time; they also track how fast you're running (your pace), how far, how many calories you've burned, and what your heart rate is. Some even monitor your body fat and give you the option of racing against yourself or competing against your best time over a particular route. Many of them also have an online and social media aspect that enables you to track your progress, map your favorite routes, and interact with fellow runners. Among the most popular GPS running watches are those from Garmin (the Forerunner series), Timex (Ironman), Nike, and Suunto.

If you don't want to spend hundreds of dollars on a watch, several free mobile apps are available, like Nike+ Running, MapMyRun, and RunKeeper, which track your distance, time, and pace and auto-sync your runs to the web so that you can compete against your pals and runners from all over the world. They can also map your route and tell you what your fastest and slowest miles were, so that you can monitor your pace.

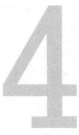

General Nutrition and Hydration

A LOT OF THOUGHT GOES INTO THE AVERAGE RUN—WHEN YOU'RE going to run and where, for how long, how fast, what you're going to wear, what music you're going to listen to, etc. Yet, many runners neglect to address the single most important thing in their planning: What are you going to eat and when?

Too often runners jump right out of bed, slip on their running shoes, grab their GPS watch or iPod, and head out on their run without so much as taking a single bite of fruit or sip of water. Maybe they're pressed for time or don't want to upset their stomach, or maybe they feel they'll lose more weight by not eating anything at all. But by skipping a pre-run meal or snack, they deprive their bodies of the energy needed to fuel their run. And the longer and harder the run, the more energy your body needs to sustain that intensity.

Eating will make you feel better pre- and post-run, according to Heidi Skolnik, a senior nutritionist for the Hospital for Special Surgery in New York City and a consultant for the New York Knicks basketball team. "From an energy standpoint, it makes a big difference. I think it's hard for people to understand that when they feel good already. They don't know how much better they could feel. So I would encourage you to take in at least 15 to 25 grams of carbohydrates before you run. It's not that much, but it might help curb that big appetite kick you get later in the day once you cool down. And you won't be as fatigued after [the run]."

As it is with so many things in running, timing is very important when it comes to nutrition and hydration. You need to get your training runs and daily workouts in sync with your eating and drinking habits so that your body can best utilize these energy sources to both bolster your runs and aid in your recovery process. This chapter is full of strategies about not only what's best to eat and drink, but also when and how much, whether you're going out to run an easy 5 miles around the neighborhood or to compete in a 10K race or a marathon.

If you haven't given much thought to nutrition or hydration before, I guarantee that you will after reading this chapter. There are all types of strategies to help you improve performance, but none is easier or more effective than learning what to put into your fuel tank, and when.

Pre-Run Nutrition

Before you head out the door for your run, make sure to fuel your tank with a small serving of carbohydrates, a component of food that supplies energy (in the form of calories) to the body. It could be a few pretzels, half a banana or energy bar, some orange juice, a sports drink, or a carb energy chew. The point is, you want to take in just enough carbs (about 15 to 25 grams) to boost your blood sugar levels and give your engine a boost. This is especially true in the morning, because when you sleep, you deplete these sugars as well as your glycogen stores, mainly in the liver.

Glycogen is a stored form of carbohydrate that is used by the body for energy. When you digest carbs, they get broken down into simple blood sugar, or glucose. This glucose is then carried through the bloodstream and deposited into your liver and muscles, where it is converted into glycogen and eventually used as energy. The more you run and train—and fuel your muscles—the greater your capacity to store this glycogen and the more energy you have to pull from your body. If you run out of these glycogen stores in your muscles and liver mid-run, then you have nowhere else to draw energy from and you're in imminent danger of bonking (hitting the wall).

As a general rule of thumb, the closer in time you are to your run, the smaller the amount of food you want to consume, says Skolnik, who was also the team nutritionist for the New York Giants football team for 18 years. If you're going to run in late morning or during your lunch hour, then have a light snack between breakfast and your workout. And make sure not to skip breakfast before you go to work. Breakfast is the most important meal of the day, and it curbs your hunger later on. You should eat a balanced breakfast consisting of complex carbs (starch), fresh fruit, and protein. Good breakfast choices include eggs, toast, berries, oatmeal, low-fat milk or yogurt, or a bagel with peanut butter.

If you prefer to run in the evening after work, then you want to have a slightly larger snack about 2 to 2½ hours beforehand to fuel your effort. A good afternoon snack might be a banana with peanut butter, low-fat yogurt with trail mix and a piece of fruit, or a granola bar with a latte. If you get busy at work or home and you miss that window, then make sure to grab a small snack about 15 to 30 minutes before your run.

Of course, you don't want to eat a large dinner and then go out for your run. For the most part, you want to leave 3 to 4 hours between a large meal and a run so that your body has enough time to fully digest the meal. You don't have to leave so much time, however, if you eat a smaller amount of food. If you plan to run in 3 hours, go ahead and have a turkey sandwich. Two hours? Then have a yogurt and some granola. An hour? A small serving of pretzels will do the trick. You're a runner, so you're always keenly aware of time—just apply it to the amount of food you eat and when you eat it as well.

Post-Run Eating

Now, if you are one of those people who run only in the evening, make sure to eat a proper, balanced meal after your workout, even if you don't get home until 8 or 9 p.m. Don't skip dinner! You need protein to help repair and build your muscles, and you need carbs to restore the energy you've lost—and to help refuel your tank for the next day's run. Some good dinner options, Skolnik says, are pasta with lean chicken and spinach, and a lean steak with broccoli and sweet potatoes.

The same holds true for breakfast. Even if you had a pre-run snack the first thing in the morning, you need to refuel after your run and get energy back in your system. Good sources of protein include eggs, low-fat cottage cheese, and low-fat yogurt. Solid carb options include bagels, whole-wheat toast, and bananas. The goal should be to consume somewhere between 400 to 600 calories after your run, says Skolnik, ideally within 30 to 60 minutes. Wait any longer and your body won't recover as well. If you have dinner or brunch plans, or you can't get to your kitchen within an hour after your run, then you should have one of the many ready-made sources of protein and carbohydrates, such as low-fat chocolate milk, a smoothie, or an energy bar or a nutrition bar. The important thing is to get something of nutritional value in your body; otherwise it won't be able to repair and rebuild itself, and you'll be more fatigued and more likely to suffer an injury on your next run.

Eating on the Run

If you plan on running for an hour or more, or at relatively moderate to high intensity, then bring fuel with you. Crushed pretzels, energy gels and chews, sports drinks, trail mix, Rice Chex, and dried fruit are all great options, as they provide you with the fuel you need to run longer and, in some instances, replenish vital electrolytes (sodium) lost while running.

Gels and chews, like those from GU, Clif, etc., are not only good sources of carbs and electrolytes but are also portable and easy to use—much easier than carrying a few bananas or oranges on your run. A sports drink also gives you the carbs and electrolytes you need, as well as the fluids. These items are convenient because they have most everything your body craves. Some runners have a hard time tolerating sports gels and drinks, however, and may get a sloshy feeling in their stomach. If you're one of them, and you prefer to drink water only, then bring some crushed pretzels along with you so that you get some sodium and carbs as well. One thing to note: Never consume too many of these gels or wash them down with a sports drink, such as Gatorade; you're only asking for stomach trouble with that combination. Make sure you take them with water.

There's no one answer to what your nutrition should be, Skolnik says. You have to experiment to see what works best and is most easily digested. For instance, don't wait until the day of a race to eat a bagel with peanut butter for the very first time, because what might work well for a friend of yours could wind up upsetting your stomach and ruining your race. Everybody is different, but one thing is for certain: You need the right balance of carbs, electrolytes, and fluids to sustain the intensity of your runs, as well as to maintain the proper body temperature. I'll talk more about the importance of electrolytes and hydration later in this chapter.

Eating for the Long Run

Throughout your training, but especially in the 24 to 48 hours leading up to a long training run or a race day, it's important that you stockpile your muscles with carbohydrate-appropriate foods (cereals, pasta, rice, bread). That said, there's no need to go crazy "carbo-loading" the day before a run by stuffing yourself with large amounts of baked ziti and pasta and neglecting other foods. If you continue to take in an adequate amount of carbs at breakfast, lunch, and dinner, then you will have already been carbo-loading and should be good to go.

Just what is an adequate amount of carbs? How much you consume depends on how far you plan on running, the intensity in which you run, and what your weight is, according to Skolnik. If you train with a low to moderate amount of intensity and your run or race is under 60 minutes, Skolnik recommends taking in 5 to 6 grams of carbohydrates daily per kilogram of body weight (your weight in pounds divided by 2.2). If, for example, you weigh 190 pounds, you want to consume roughly 475 grams of carbs per day (190 ÷ 2.2 x 5.5), or about 1,900 kilocalories. If the run is more than 60 minutes long and you train at low to moderate intensity, then Skolnik suggests you consume a slightly higher number of carbohydrates (6 to 10 grams per kilogram of body weight). For those training at a higher intensity (i.e., speedwork, hill repeats) or for a long-distance race, such as a marathon, she suggests taking in 7 to 10 grams or even more per kilogram of body weight. For that same 190-pound runner, that could be as many as 850 grams of carbs or more per day.

The night before a long run or a marathon, Skolnik recommends that you "top off the tank." Before you go to bed, have a carb-rich snack such as a serving of pretzels, a bowl of cereal, or half a bagel with peanut butter.

"When you sleep, you go through your blood sugar because you're feeding your brain and feeding your kidneys, lungs, and heart," she says. "All of those things are working while you sleep. Your muscles haven't depleted, but your blood sugar has dropped, and you've used your liver glycogen. When you eat before you go to sleep, you're giving yourself a little edge in that you're not as depleted as you'd be if you didn't eat after, say, 7 p.m."

On the morning of a long run, follow the guidelines we established earlier, eating smaller amounts of food the closer in time you are to the start of your run. If it's a marathon and you're waking up some 5 or 6 hours before the start of the race, then have yourself a good breakfast and then a carb-friendly snack 30 to 45 minutes before the start of the race.

Running and Dieting

Anyone who's ever trained for a distance event knows how difficult it is to lose weight while in training. When you're running 30-, 40-, or 50-plus miles per week, it's very easy to overload on carbs because that's what your body craves—your fuel tank is in constant need of being replenished to energize your runs. Many runners also view their training as an excuse to eat whatever they want, whenever they want, thinking that they can't possibly gain any weight with all the running they're doing. But the reality is that some runners might see a gain of a few pounds while in training, especially during the 3-week taper preceding the race, when their weekly mileage starts to decline.

It's extremely hard to lose weight and still get the proper amount of carbo-hydrates your body needs to log all those miles in training, which is why I rec-ommend that if you're going to use running as a means to complement a diet, you do so prior to beginning training. Running can be a highly effective way to lose weight and keep it off, but not when you're preparing your body to run 13.1 or 26.2 miles.

Those of you who are trying to lose weight and are not in training don't need to change your diet all that much. You just want to make sure you're taking in the appropriate amount of carbs before, during, and after your runs, so that you're fueling your runs and aiding your recovery. Eating half a bagel with some peanut butter (roughly 350 calories) 30 minutes before your run is not going to make you fat, because you're going to burn that many calories and more during your workout. Your regular diet should include an adequate amount of carbs at every meal, along with proteins and healthy fats. If you need a late-morning or mid-afternoon pick-me-up, then snack on fruit, yogurt, or nuts and skip the muffins, pastries, chips, and candy.

The Female Athlete Triad

Recent studies indicate that weight loss can hurt your bone health (i.e., it can lower bone density), and we know that women tend to be on a diet more often than men. We also know that women have less muscle and bone mass than men and that their daily calorie needs are fewer. Therefore, female runners need to be very smart about their diet and make sure that they're getting an adequate amount of daily carbohydrates, healthy fats, and most important, protein and calcium.

Calcium is crucial to maintaining strong bone health. This mineral is absorbed readily by our bodies and stored in our bones and teeth, much like glycogen is stored in our muscles and liver. As we age, however, our bodies draw more on these stores to aid normal functioning of the nervous and cardiovascular systems. In other words, the body takes out much more than it puts back into our bones. That explains why most Americans—about 50 percent, according to recent studies—are calcium-deficient. Postmenopausal women are even more susceptible to a calcium deficiency, since the estrogen levels that help to protect the bones from calcium loss are depleted.

The recommended dietary allowance (RDA) of calcium for women ages 19 to 50 is 1,000 milligrams per day; for women 51 and older, this increases to 1,200 milligrams per day. Good sources of calcium include dairy products such as cheese (Romano, Swiss, cheddar), yogurt (about 400 milligrams per cup), and low-fat milk (300 milligrams per cup); calcium-fortified orange juice (290 milligrams per cup); raw tofu processed with calcium (435 milligrams per ½ cup); and cooked spinach (120 milligrams per ½ cup).

Decreased bone density, or osteoporosis, is associated with one of the three interrelated conditions that make up the Female Athlete Triad, or Triad. The others are eating disorders (anorexia, bulimia, or other unhealthy weight-control behaviors) and amenorrhea (the absence of a woman's menstrual period). This syndrome is often seen in female athletes who carry very little body fat, such as runners. In many instances, the athlete is deliberately trying to lose weight; or, between working, socializing, training, and perhaps raising children, she is simply not getting the fuel she needs.

"Either way, you create this energy deficit, which really drains your body," Skolnik says. "Your body begins to shut down nonessential functions like getting your period. It's not getting the nutrients it needs, including protein and calcium, and so you're not building proper bone density."

If this goes on long enough, you become more vulnerable to stress fractures and early osteoporosis. Men also have to deal with decreasing levels of hormones (testosterone) as they get older, which results in a loss of muscle mass and bone strength as well. Therefore, it's important that they get enough protein and calcium in their diet. And since men have more muscle mass and thus burn more calories than their female counterparts, it's vital that they consume more carbohydrates—especially runners who need them to maintain their glycogen and energy levels.

Anti-inflammatory Foods

Starting in the 1980s, there was evidence that certain foods could help combat inflammation, and that body of evidence has only grown in recent years. This is big news for runners, especially those who log a lot of miles and walk a thin line between being healthy and being injured. Their diets need to be as rich in these anti-inflammatory foods as they are in energy foods (i.e., carbs), because it's just as important to help the body repair from a run as it is to fuel it for one.

Today's modern diet is not helping the average runner. It's filled with processed foods containing high-fructose corn syrup, preservatives (hydrogenated oil or trans fats), and saturated fats (animal fats, cooking oils), all of which increase the general level of inflammation in the body, making it harder for you to recover from your runs. These readily available foods lack the essential vitamins, minerals, fiber, and antioxidants your body needs to rebuild itself, and they can trigger your body's natural defense system to respond in much the same way as it would to a wound or a life-threatening situation. And that's not all: The consumption of trans fats is known to increase your risk for a number of degenerative chronic ailments, including coronary heart disease, stroke, and diabetes. It does this by raising levels of "bad" LDL (low-density-lipoprotein) cholesterol and lowering levels of "good" HDL (high-density-lipoprotein) cholesterol.

What you should do is fill your diet with a lot of the same foods our forebears ate hundreds of years ago—unprocessed foods rich in vitamins, antioxidants, omega-3 essential fatty acids (EFAs), and fiber. These foods include brightly colored fruits and vegetables high in carotenoids and bioflavonoids (blueberries, raspberries, red grapes, mangoes, kiwi, kale, spinach, broccoli), nuts (walnuts, macadamia nuts), whole grains (brown rice, oats), and cold-water fish (salmon, tuna, bass). The latter is an abundant source of two very effective omega-3 unsaturated fatty acids, known as eicosapentaenoic acid (EPA) and docosahexaenoic acid (DHA). These oils have been shown to reduce the risk of blood clotting and arterial plaque buildup, and they are extremely effective in fighting inflammation. One study conducted by the University of Washington showed that people who consume two or more servings of fish rich in omega-3 each week are 40 percent less likely to develop arthritis later in life.

Omega-3 EFAs appear to turn off inflammatory reactions when the body no longer needs them, whereas omega-6 EFAs, which are found in red meat and many animal fats and vegetable oils, promote inflammation. These oils are not only used to fry foods but are also added to most processed foods, microwavable foods, frozen foods, and candy bars. The ideal ratio of omega-6 to omega-3 fats is roughly 2:1, but in today's modern diet, the average ratio is more than 20:1, which is not good for long-term health.

I advise all of my patients to follow an anti-inflammatory diet that's relatively low in calories but extremely high in the vitamins, minerals, and nutrients we need to sustain our health, including protein. Obviously, runners need more calories to fuel their training, but by eliminating trans fats altogether, limiting the amount of saturated fats they consume, and gravitating to foods that help fight inflammation, they stand a much better chance of staying healthy and on their feet.

Avoiding the 100-Meter Dash (to the Bathroom)

It happens to a lot of runners: They're 4 or 5 miles into their morning run and feeling great when suddenly, they're doing their best Usain Bolt imitation and sprinting to the nearest bathroom. For those who run in places like Central Park, where restrooms abound, it's a minor inconvenience. But for others who are miles away from home or a bathroom, it's not a lot of fun. And it can completely ruin your race experience. In fact, for many runners, their greatest fear about running a half- or full marathon is not the distance, but rather about having to go to the bathroom during the race. This can be very uncomfortable and stressful, and it can cost you a lot of precious time if you're trying to establish a personal best or break a time barrier, such as 3 or 4 hours.

If you're one of these people who experiences gastrointestinal distress from time to time when you run, you're not alone. According to Skolnik, 25 to 50 percent of endurance athletes can experience some abdominal cramping, nausea, diarrhea, or flatulence during or after exercise. The major reason for this is that while you're running, blood flow is diverted away from the intestines to your muscles, which disrupts normal gastrointestinal activity and can lead to loose bowel movements. The up-and-down motion associated with running also can stir the bowels, causing waste material to pass through the intestines at a faster rate. Other common causes of gastrointestinal distress include dehydration, irritable bowel syndrome, and lactose intolerance. If you find that the problem arises only during races, then it could be anxiety related.

From a dietary standpoint, the best way to eliminate frequent trips to the bathroom is to experiment with consuming different foods and beverages before you run, so you get a good sense of what you can eat and what makes you go to the bathroom. Avoiding high-fiber foods such as beans, nuts, dark chocolate, and flaxseed and those with bran (whole-grain breads, rice, oats) before you run is also a good idea.

Once you discover a few foods that are runner-friendly, then you want to practice eating these foods at those times of the day that match up with your regular running schedule or the time of your race.

"You've got to learn what's best for you," Skolnik says. "If you always like to run first thing in the morning, but you've never run at 10 a.m. [the approximate start time of the New York City Marathon], you should practice that, because the delay from the time you wake up till you run is several hours. You may want to try getting up at 5 a.m. and running at 10, so you know what it's like to have oatmeal, two eggs and a glass of juice at 5 in the morning, and then a little bagel with peanut butter at 8:30."

Proper Hydration Strategies

One of the leading causes of running injuries is dehydration. According to Skolnik, nearly half the people who walk out the door in the morning to run or go work out are already dehydrated. They may have had a few sips of coffee, but their water tank is about as dry as the Sahara Desert. Just as your body needs carbohydrates for energy, it must have fluids to fuel the proper contraction and relaxation of the muscles so that they can perform most efficiently. If you're running low on these fluids, then these muscles become more susceptible to strains and cramps.

A big part of the problem is that people wait until they're thirsty to drink, and that's a bad idea, since part of being dehydrated is that you lose your thirst; thus, you have a hard time recognizing when you are thirsty. "You need to be a little ahead of your thirst," says Skolnik, who recommends treating hydration much like you do eating, and planning a schedule around what you're going to drink before, during, and after your runs.

How much fluid you consume depends on a number of things, including your weight, the duration of the run, the temperature outside, and how much you sweat. If you're going on a short, non-intense run (i.e., less than an hour), you should consume roughly 6 to 8 ounces of water before you head out the door. If you're going on a more intense run, such as a 5K or 10K race, or if it's hot and humid outside, then you should also consume a few ounces of a sports drink. These drinks provide both carbs and electrolytes, including sodium, which the body sweats out during intense runs. For a longer run, you should drink 8 to 16 ounces of water or a sports drink an hour before your run and another 4 to 8 ounces as you walk out the door. If it's unusually hot outside or you're a larger-size runner, then you may want to drink a bit more. Just make sure you're not taking in too much water and depleting your body of sodium, which can lead to a dangerous, sometimes life-threatening condition known as hyponatremia.

Determining Your Sweat Rate

As for hydrating on the run, a good rule of thumb is to drink 6 to 10 ounces of water every 15 minutes, mixing some electrolytes in there, too, when the weather is warm and the run is long in duration. Some people may need to consume more, others less, but the idea is to replace the amount of sweat your body lost, within 2 percent.

If you're not sure how much that is, Skolnik recommends weighing yourself before and after your run and taking note of how much weight you lost. Then add back in the amount of water and sports drink you ingested during the run to return your body to your pre-run weight and determine your average sweat rate. For example, if you weighed 160 pounds before the run and 158 afterward, then you lost approximately 2 pounds of water weight, a sweat loss of 32 ounces. But if you consumed roughly 24 ounces of fluids during the run, you must figure in that amount, which brings your sweat loss to 56 ounces. Divide that over the course of 2 hours, and it becomes roughly 28 ounces of sweat per hour. Therefore, you would need to drink approximately 7 ounces of water or sports drink every 15 minutes to stay properly hydrated.

Sports Drinks and Electrolytes

The longer your run and the hotter it is outside, the greater your risk of dehydration, because your body has to sweat more to keep itself cool. The main ingredient in sweat is sodium, which is why you need to replenish your body frequently with electrolytes as well as water. Electrolytes are salts and minerals that are responsible for transmitting electrical signals in the body, in particular to your muscles. If you don't get enough of these electrolytes, then these signals are weakened and your muscles start to perform sluggishly. You are also at a greater risk of cramping, which no runner ever wants to experience, especially during a race. If you're properly hydrated, then your body is more heat-acclimated and your sweat has less sodium, thus reducing your chances of cramping.

Sports drinks and energy gels are your best sources for electrolytes, as they include not only sodium but also carbohydrates to fuel your muscles. If you're going to consume several gels during your run in lieu of a sports drink, make sure you add a fluid component by taking them with water. Many runners find that these gels easier to carry around with them than, say, a 16-ounce bottle of Gatorade, but they can upset your stomach if you don't chase them with water.

On longer runs, it's better to drink smaller amounts of fluids more frequently than large amounts all at once, since the body has an easier time absorbing liquid in small doses, Skolnik says. Runners should consider drinking 4 to 8 ounces of a sports drink every 20 minutes on these bigger runs, alternating between these drinks and water every other mile or stop—especially if the race they're competing in provides both.

Post-Run Hydration

The very first thing most runners do after a workout or a race is to head straight for the water fountain or table. They don't need any convincing when it comes to getting something to drink. Many consume just water alone, however, and forget to take in the appropriate amount of carbohydrates, electrolytes, and protein their body needs to repair and rebuild itself and to put energy back in their system.

Ready-made smoothies and other drinks that contain all three of these energy sources are available. One of the best is low-fat chocolate milk; a 16-ounce bottle of Nestlé Nesquik low-fat chocolate milk has 50 grams of carbohydrates, 16 gram of protein, 840 milligrams of potassium (another important source of electrolytes), and 320 milligrams of sodium. The sooner you consume one of these drinks after a race or workout—Skolnik recommends within 30 to 60 minutes of your run—the more quickly you'll recover.

Coffee, Energy Drinks, and Other Stimulants

In 2012, energy drinks Red Bull and Monster combined for more than $5.5 billion in sales. The top-selling energy shot, 5-Hour Energy, did just short of $900 million in sales. These drinks contain high levels of caffeine and sugar—stacked with other stimulants such as taurine, ginseng, guarana, and ginkgo biloba—to give you an energy and alertness boost similar to that from one or two cups of coffee. According to a 2012 *Consumer Reports* article on energy drinks, a 2-ounce shot of Extra Strength 5-Hour Energy has as much caffeine (242 milligrams) as a tall (12-ounce) cup of Starbucks brewed coffee.

While a small amount of caffeine can help your physical performance, consuming too much can have very negative and dangerous side effects, such as elevating your blood pressure and accelerating your heart rate. Caffeine is also a diuretic and can contribute to dehydration. Therefore, if you must have your morning cup of joe, limit it to one 8-ounce cup and make sure to consume at least an equal amount of water before you head out the door. If you swear by 5-Hour Energy or one of those other energy drinks, drink a half serving instead of a whole bottle or can. You don't need that much caffeine. If you feel the least bit jittery or full of adrenaline, then stay away from caffeine and substitute orange juice or a sports drink full of carbs and electrolytes in its place.

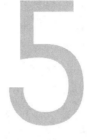

Speed Is Strength in Disguise

THE FIRST QUESTION YOU NEED TO ASK YOURSELF WHEN YOU SIGN UP for a race is "What's my goal?" If you're running in your very first race and your goal is simply to finish, which it should be, then you need to set up your training to meet that goal. You'll want to run a lot of long, slow miles so that you learn how to endure and stay on your feet for several hours. You needn't concern yourself with speed. You should run at a comfortable pace and train at a comfortable pace. Get your first race under your belt before you start worrying about your time.

If, however, you're a 4½-hour marathoner who wants to run a sub-4-hour marathon, or you're trying to shave 15 minutes off your time to qualify for the Boston Marathon, then you'll have to train differently. You'll want to add some sport-specific elements to your training regimen, such as strength training and intervals (speedwork). To achieve peak performance, you must train both anaerobically and aerobically, starting with anaerobic training (weight lifting, sprinting, jumping) and working toward the aerobic side (jogging, swimming, cycling) of the spectrum. In the middle of this spectrum are your intervals and cross-training workouts, which are a mix of anaerobic and aerobic. Hit all three levels of the continuum and you'll get your speed up and improve your time.

Anaerobic exercise is key. Aerobic means "with oxygen" and anaerobic means "without oxygen." Anaerobic exercise is intense enough to produce lactic acid, whereas aerobic exercise is not. When you train aerobically, your heart and lungs deliver oxygen-rich blood to your muscles, which they use as energy (along with glucose) to help sustain a low to moderate level of exertion over a longer stretch of time. This is how you'll spend the vast majority of your training, running aerobically at a smooth, comfortable pace. When you train anaerobically, there's a temporary shortage of oxygen being delivered to your muscles, and your primary source of fuel is stored glycogen. Lactic acid begins to accumulate in your blood, and your muscles start to become very fatigued and sore, which is why most anaerobic activity is short in duration—up to 2 minutes, at most.

With increased anaerobic exercise, your body becomes better equipped to handle this lactic acid and perform at a higher intensity without becoming fatigued as quickly. As a result, you're able to increase your aerobic endurance potential or VO_2 max.

Strength training is the best form of anaerobic exercise, since it involves very short, intense bursts of muscular activity. Sprinting is another. Yet runners often overlook strength training as they prepare for a race because they either don't have the time for it or think it's detrimental to their training (i.e., that it leads to sore muscles). Another camp of runners thinks that running alone will give them all the strength they need to tackle 26.2 miles on race day. That's true, to some degree: If you're doing your training runs in Central Park, you're running a lot of hills, and in the process, you're building strength in your quads and glutes. You're also strengthening your aerobic capacity and ability to run easier over a longer distance. Through additional strength training, however, you'll maximize the anaerobic effect and build even more lean muscle and speed.

As I noted in chapter 1, speed is strength in disguise, meaning that you'll run faster and more efficiently if you supplement your long, slow distance runs with short, very intense anaerobic workouts. By strength training two or three times per week, you'll build more lean muscle mass and, as a result, be able to recruit more muscle fibers to help power your legs when your glycogen reserves are getting low. This is critical when you're at mile 22 of the marathon and it's getting harder and harder to turn your legs over and sustain your desired pace.

Weight training has several other benefits. For one, it helps strengthen the muscles and muscle-tendon junctions in your lower extremities. These are your primary shock absorbers when you run, and the stronger they are, the more cushion they provide for your body. Strength training also increases bone density, reducing the risk of osteoporosis and stress fractures. Bone is a live tissue and constantly breaking down and building up—strength training helps facilitate this repairing phase. From a performance standpoint, stronger muscles have a greater workload potential. They're able to carry your body weight over longer distances, thus improving your endurance.

Stronger Muscles Also Help You over the Short Haul

"When you're doing speedwork, you're loading a little differently," says Joseph Feinberg, MD, physiatrist in chief at the Hospital for Special Surgery in New York and the team physician for St. Peter's University in Jersey City, New Jersey—and a runner for more than 40 years. "It's faster, and there's a greater force, so you need to have good eccentric control of the muscles. If you don't, then over time you're going to be excessively loading other structures. You want your muscles to develop so that you can handle that."

"Eccentric" means that the muscle under tension is lengthening as it's contracting. Also known as negative training, eccentric training is said to create superior strength in the muscle, as compared to concentric loading—when the muscle is shortening. If you're performing a leg press, the eccentric portion of the exercise is when you're lowering the weight and bringing your knees toward you, not when you're pushing the weight and extending your legs. Many people get these confused. The hamstring muscles are actually lengthening as you return the weight to the starting position. Perhaps the simplest way to remember it is that the eccentric movement occurs when you're trying to control or slow down the action, and you're moving the weight with gravity.

Perhaps the best reason of all to incorporate strength exercises into your training regimen is that Father Time necessitates it. At about the age of 40, you start to lose approximately 1 percent muscle mass per year. This is largely due to a steady decline in hormones—testosterone in men and estrogen in women. Your tissues also begin to lose water—about 1 percent per year—which means your muscles and tendons begin to lose their elasticity, putting greater stresses on your joints and other weight-bearing structures. You're not going to be able to reverse either trend, but you can significantly slow them down and minimize their impact with strength training.

In this chapter, we're going to look at anaerobic training. The following 15 strength-training exercises are geared specifically toward runners and can be done easily at home without much in the way of equipment. You'll be using your own body weight for the majority of the exercises, placing a strong emphasis on the eccentric, or slow-down, phase of each movement, which places the maximum load on the muscles and muscle-tendon junctions being worked.

I recommend that you find the time for two 30-minute strength-training sessions per week. Think about it: That's 1 hour per week, or about the time it takes you to complete a midweek training run. If it's easier, incorporate a couple of shorter workouts (15 minutes) into your training regimen. Never strength-train before you run; save these sessions for your rest/recovery days or for after your runs. Exercises such as calf raises (page 61), standing leg kicks (page 63), and knee lifts (page 65) go well with that post-run smoothie. Always make sure your muscles are warm before you perform any strength-training exercises, and remember to brace yourself with your abdominals (abs in) to provide greater stability, as well as to protect your spine.

Lower-Body Exercises

Running is a one-legged activity, which means the weight-bearing muscles, tendons, and joints in your lower body take on more forces and loads than they would if you were walking. In fact, the force exerted on each foot as it strikes the ground can be as much as three to five times your body weight. As a result, it's very important that you keep these weight-bearing muscles (calves, hamstrings, quadriceps, glutes) strong, so that you not only endure longer but also avoid common injuries (stress fractures, muscle strains, tendinosis) associated with these impact stresses. Here are a few lower-body exercises designed to make that impact a little easier.

Double- and Single-Leg Calf Raises

✤ Your calves are responsible for extending the ankle and lifting your feet up off the ground. They also have such a low nerve supply that they need to be trained harder than all the other muscles in your lower body. There simply aren't enough nerve impulses to stimulate the muscles into activity, which is why they need to be strengthened. Here's how. Stand on the edge of a step with only your toes and the balls of your feet in contact with the step. Push up off your toes, raising both heels several inches above the step.

✤ Slowly return your heels to the same height as the step (not below it), and continue this up-and-down motion for 10 repetitions. Complete three sets of 10 reps. You can increase the resistance and intensity of this exercise by holding a pair of light dumbbells in each hand or by working one calf at a time. To perform a single-leg calf raise, secure one foot behind the other and push up off your toes on your standing foot, lifting your heel as high as you can. Use the wall for balance, and try to keep your ankle, knee, and hip on the standing leg in alignment as you press forward on your toes.

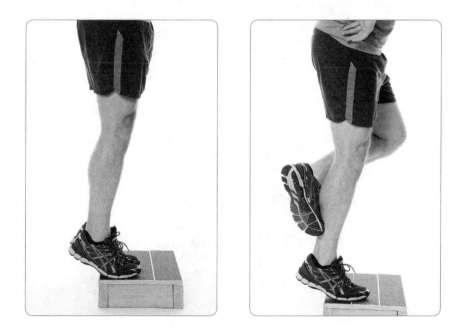

Double-Leg Toe Raises

✤ Weak tibialis anterior and calf muscles are often responsible for a painful condition known as shin splints, which is typically felt in the connective tissue along or behind the tibia. Performing these toe raises on a regular basis will help prevent shin splints from recurring, while also improving your toe liftoff when running. Stand up straight with your feet approximately shoulder-width apart, and raise your toes slowly up off the floor and toward the ceiling while keeping your heels on the floor.

✤ At the top of the movement, hold for a count of three before returning to the starting position. Perform three sets of 10 reps to help strengthen the muscles at the front of your lower leg, in particular the tibialis anterior muscle, which connects to your shinbone. (Note: To work these muscles even harder, lift your toes while standing on only one leg.)

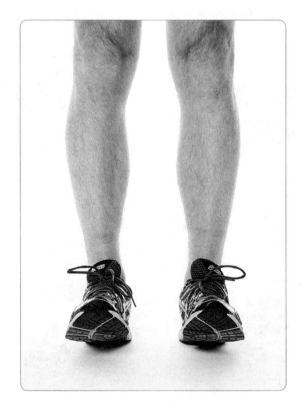

Standing Leg Kicks

✢ This is a great exercise to do after a run and on your rest/recovery days. Stand up straight with your arms extended diagonally out in front of you to help with balance. Lift your right foot about an inch off the ground and kick it directly out to the side about 6 to 12 inches.

✢ Immediately return your right foot back to center, and repeat in a back-and-forth, fluid motion, like a windshield wiper. Keep your movements very small. Perform 50 to 100 single-leg kicks on each leg to strengthen the hip abductor muscles and iliotibial band on your standing leg. To add a level of difficulty, either increase the number of reps or kick the leg out at a slower, more deliberate pace, which will force your standing leg to work harder to maintain proprioception, or balance. Make sure to line up the center of your forehead, chest, and navel with the inside of your standing ankle as you move the kicking leg away from the center of your body, as this will prevent your lower body from swaying. The hip abductor muscles play a critical role in helping to stabilize the pelvis and maintain good posture. These muscles are very prone to fatigue, so the stronger they are, the longer you'll endure.

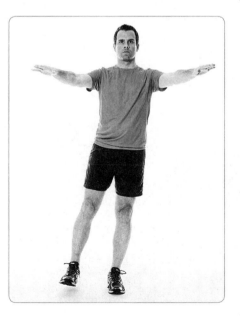

Single-Leg Lifts, Lying Down

✤ Lie on your back with your arms out to your sides at a 90-degree angle, perpendicular to your chest. Bend one knee so your thigh is at about a 45-degree angle, then raise the other leg up and down—fast on the way up, slow on the way down—keeping the toes pointed upward.

✤ Lift your leg only as high as the opposite leg's thigh (so it's parallel to the thigh), and lower it until the heel is approximately an inch off the floor. Move the leg up and down for a count of 10 deep breaths in and out, and then repeat with the opposite leg. Draw your abdominals in toward your spine to provide additional support, and feel as if you're pushing your lower back into the floor as you raise each leg. The lowering, eccentric phase of this exercise really targets the lower abdominals while strengthening your hip flexors, quadriceps, and hamstrings.

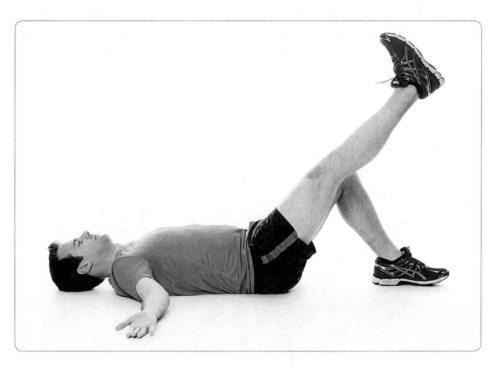

Knee Lifts

✤ This strengthening exercise is best performed after your training runs, when your legs are fatigued and your balance is shaky at best. Stand tall with your feet about shoulder-width apart, and march straight ahead for approximately 30 feet, or 10 meters, slowly bringing your knees and thighs up toward your chest.

✤ At the top of the motion, your thighs should be parallel to the ground, or 90 degrees to your body. After 30 feet, turn around and march in the other direction at the same slow speed, again lifting your knees high off the ground. Perform 3 reps at 30 feet. At first you'll find it very difficult to lift your knees so high and still maintain your balance. Part of that is the slow pace in which you want to perform the movements. This is a great exercise to build strength in your quadriceps and hip flexor muscles, which are responsible for extending the knees as well as pulling your knees up (i.e., flexing the hip joints). These muscles are very important in the swing phase of your running gait cycle. The quads also help to stabilize the knee, making you less susceptible to injury.

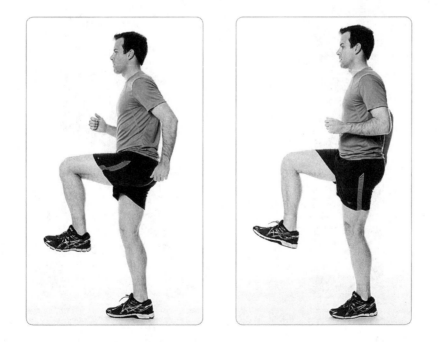

Monster Walks

✤ Loop a TheraBand, Versa-Loop, or other resistance band around your ankles so that it's nice and taut. Take a shoulder-width stance with your knees slightly bent, elbows at your sides, and hands in front of you—similar to a wrestling pose or that of a monster. Engage your abs and walk slowly from side to side, taking five small steps to your right and five to your left to complete one set.

✤ Make sure to use your glutes as you step outward and to keep the band tight at all times. Perform three sets to really fire your glutes and hip abductor muscles. (Note: The wider you step, the more you work the hip abductors.) Walk forward and backward for three sets of five steps as well, again taking small steps and controlling the motion with your glutes. Draw your abs in for additional stability.

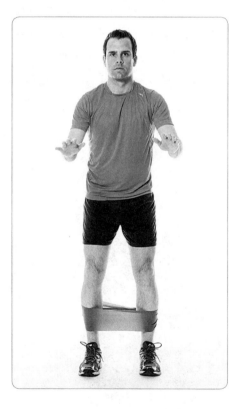 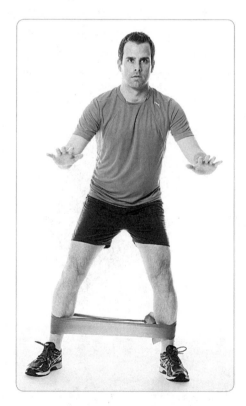

Modified Single-Leg Squat

✛ This is a great exercise for building strength in your glutes, as well as in your hamstrings and quadriceps, and it doesn't put nearly as much stress on the knees as a regular squat. Stand on one leg, suspending the other foot behind the standing calf. Extend your arms out in front of you, at about a 45-degree angle, to help with balance. Initiate the squat by pushing your hips back and sitting your weight into your heel. Lower yourself only a few inches toward the floor, so there's about a 5- to 10-degree angle to your thigh.

✛ Press back up through your heel and return to the starting position. Perform three sets of 10 repetitions. Several recent studies have linked weak glutes and/or hip abductors to two very common running injuries: iliotibial band syndrome (ITBS) and patellofemoral pain syndrome, also known as runner's knee. Weak glutes lead to muscle imbalances that can impact not only your knees but also your hips and lower back. The stronger your glutes, the less susceptible you are to incurring these injuries. The glutes, along with your hamstrings, play a major role in extending your hips and propelling your body forward.

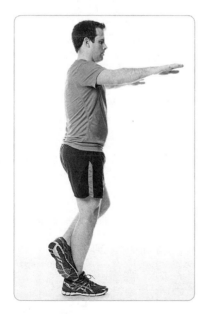 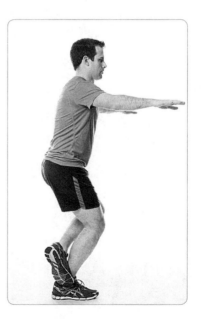

Full-Body/Core Exercises

The following exercises work your entire body and, in particular, your core, a collection of muscles and tendons that make up your body's midsection. While your lower body is the primary engine in running and your upper body the secondary, or booster, engine, the core is the conduit that harnesses the power of these two engines, lifting your feet off the ground and propelling your body forward. It transfers power from the ground up (your legs to your arms) and vice versa, creating more speed. Your core also helps stabilize your body, much like the metal beams that make up the central support system of a skyscraper. The stronger your core, the easier it is to maintain your center of gravity, and the more efficient you'll be.

> While your lower body is the primary engine in running and your upper body the secondary, or booster, engine, the core is the conduit that harnesses the power of these two engines, lifting your feet off the ground and propelling your body forward.

Plank

✢ Position yourself facedown in a plank position so that the vast majority of your weight is supported by your forearms. Your feet and elbows should be shoulder-width apart and your elbows directly underneath your shoulders. Draw your abdominals in and raise your hips and torso off the floor as one unit, maintaining a straight line from your shoulders to your ankles.

✢ Squeeze your glutes to provide additional support; do not allow your hips to sag toward the floor. Hold this position for 30 seconds, then repeat twice more. As the exercise becomes easier, increase the time to 45 seconds and then 60. To make it even more intense, lift one leg off the ground as you hold the pose. This exercise targets the deepest of the abdominals, the transverse abdominals, as well as the quads, glutes, lower back, and shoulders. It's a great exercise to help stabilize the spine.

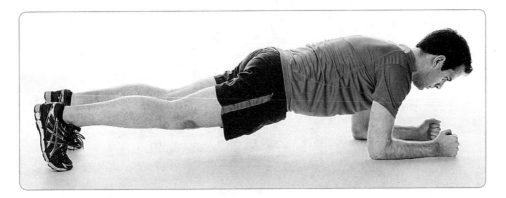

Standing Tree Pose

✤ Stand nice and tall with your arms at your sides and your feet positioned just inside your shoulders. Bring your right foot up and rest it against the inside of your left calf muscle, forming a figure-four with your legs. Inhale fully as you sweep your arms up above your head, gently pressing the sole of your right foot into your left leg as you reach for the sky.

✤ Exhale slowly and take nine more deep breaths in and out, looking to your core to help stabilize you. Try to maintain a straight line between your forehead, sternum, navel, and standing ankle as you hold the pose. Return to the starting position and repeat on the other leg. If you want to add a level of difficulty, close your eyes as you hold each pose. This exercise will help you improve proprioception on the standing leg, as well as strengthen your hip abductors, glutes, quads, and calves.

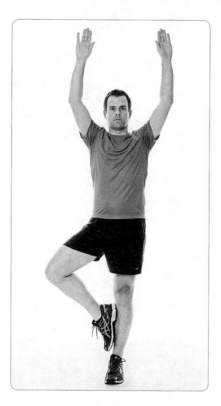

Abdominal Crunch

✣ Lie on your back with your hands behind your head, both knees bent, and feet flat on the floor. Draw your abdominals in toward your spine so that your lower back rests on the floor—you should feel as if you're trying to crack a peanut shell with your lower back. Slowly raise one leg until it's parallel to the thigh on the other leg. Next, tuck your chin into your chest and then slowly raise your head and shoulders until your shoulders are completely off the floor. Fix your gaze on your navel as you crunch your abdominals between your rib cage and pelvis.

✣ Hold for a count of 10 deep breaths in and out, then switch legs. Repeat twice more to work these important pelvic stabilizers. Raising one leg off the floor also helps isolate the lower abs.

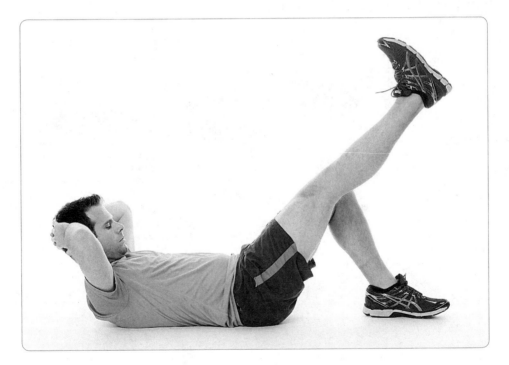

Bird Dog

✤ Assume a position on all fours, with your weight distributed evenly on your hands and knees. Inhale slowly as you raise one leg and extend it behind you, parallel to the floor. Then lift the opposite arm and extend it forward, keeping your hips and shoulders parallel to the floor. Your neck and upward leg should form one long, continuous line.

✤ Also, it's very important that the hand on your stabilizing arm be directly underneath your shoulder, and the stabilizing knee directly underneath your hip. Exhale slowly, and continue to hold for two additional deep breaths in and out. Return to the starting position and repeat on the other leg and arm, completing 10 reps on each side. This is a great strengthening and stability exercise for the glutes, as well as for your abdominal and lower back muscles.

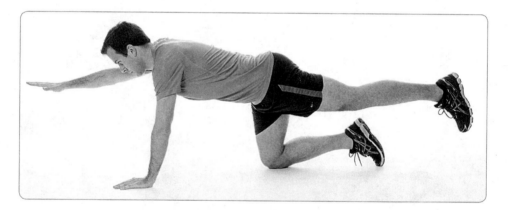

Upper-Body Exercises

Back when Tom Fleming was running 160 miles per week and challenging the world's best marathoners, he was also doing 750 push-ups per day. At 6-foot-1 and 159 pounds, Fleming was bigger than most of his competition. But while the extra weight proved to be a disadvantage, the strength training he did for his arms and upper body proved very beneficial. Fleming believes that the more upper-body strength a runner has, the more efficient the arm motion is and the faster he or she will be able to churn over those legs.

"Think about it: What's the most tired part of your body after a marathon? It's certainly not your arms. It's your legs," Fleming says. "If you strengthen your arms, you might not be so tired in the legs. Your arms dictate what happens below your waist, with your legs. They dictate what your speed is. I rarely will say to one of my athletes, 'Move your legs faster.' I will say, 'Move your arms faster.'"

Since your legs and core muscles serve as your primary engine in running, and your upper body is the secondary, or booster booster, engine that keeps the lower half running smoothly, you've got to have strength in both. With this in mind, here are a few good upper-body workouts for you to try.

> The more upper-body strength runners have, the more efficient their arm motion is and the faster they will be able to churn over those legs.

Push-ups

✤ Position yourself on your hands and your toes with your hands flat on the floor, slightly wider than shoulder-width apart. Your body should form a straight line from your head down to your ankles. Engage your abs by pulling them in toward your tailbone, and keep them engaged for the duration of the exercise. Slowly lower your entire body until your chest gently touches the floor, pause for an instant, and then push your chest and body up off the floor until you reach the starting position.

✤ (Hint: Imagine there's a string attached to your belly button and it's pulling you up toward the ceiling.) Pause for a second, and then repeat. You should feel as if your core is in control of the entire movement. Do not allow your hips to sag toward the floor, and keep your back as straight as possible throughout the exercise. Work up to three sets of 10 reps to strengthen your triceps and chest muscles, as well as your shoulders and core.

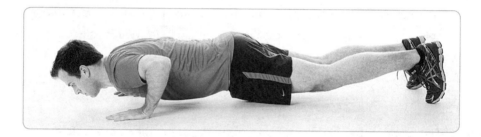

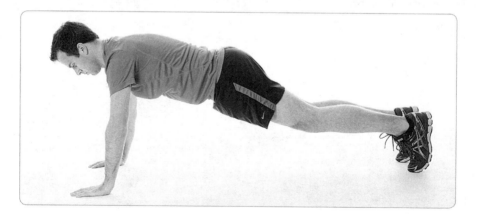

Wall Push-ups

✤ If you have difficulty performing push-ups on the floor, try a modified version standing up, using a wall for resistance. Stand facing a wall, and place your hands flat on the wall at chest level, slightly wider than shoulder-width apart. Walk your feet away from the wall until your heels are just off the ground. This is your starting position.

✤ From here, lean your body toward the wall, maintaining a straight line from your ankles to your shoulders. (Tighten your abs to maintain this neutral spine position.) Stop when your chest is about a foot from the wall, and then push your upper body back away from the wall until you reach the starting position. That's one repetition. Perform three sets of 10 reps, slowly controlling the motion as you push back from the wall.

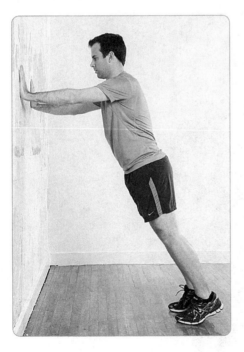 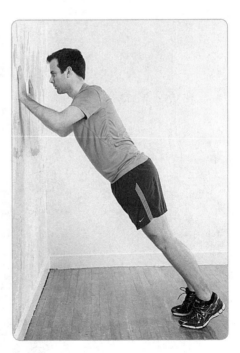

Dumbbell Hammer Curl

✧ Grasp a 5- to 15-pound dumbbell in each hand and hold them so that your palms are facing you. Stand up tall with your feet shoulder-width apart, and curl each dumbbell up until your thumbs point to each shoulder.

✧ Slowly return the dumbbells back to the starting position and repeat, keeping your elbows in front of your hips at all times. This slow-moving eccentric phase puts the maximum load on the muscle and muscle-tendon junction as they're being lengthened. Every exercise you do, including the push-up (see previous pages), should be performed in a similar fashion—quick up, slow down. Perform three sets of 10 reps to help strengthen your biceps and the muscles of the forearm, in particular the brachioradialis, which acts to flex the forearm at the elbow while you're running. This bent position is how most athletes carry their arms while they're running.

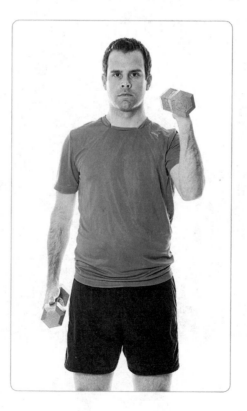

Dumbbell Hammer to Overhead

✤ This is an extension of the previous exercise, but has the additional benefit of working both your core and shoulder (deltoid) muscles. With your palms facing each other, curl both dumbbells up to your shoulders, again keeping your elbows in front of your hips. Pause for an instant, and then press both dumbbells straight up toward the ceiling.

✤ At this point, both dumbbells should be directly above your shoulders, and your arms straight. Lower both dumbbells slowly back to your shoulders, and then return them to the starting position (at your sides). Perform three sets of 10 reps.

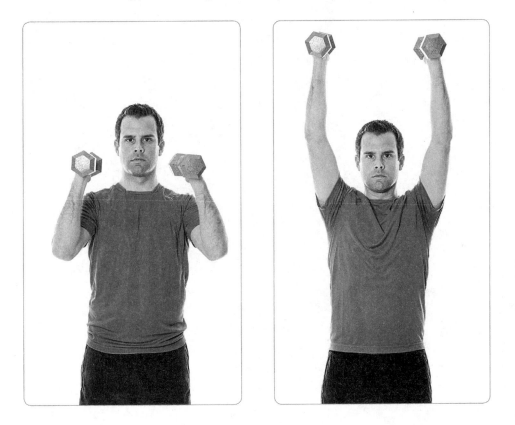

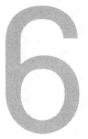

Sport-Specific Training and Interval Training

RECREATIONAL RUNNING IS, BY DEFINITION, AN AEROBIC EXERCISE, because you're using oxygen (in addition to carbohydrates) for energy and not producing lactic acid. In an aerobic state, your heart rate remains fairly low and the pace is relaxed and easy. Not so with anaerobic exercise, which gets your heart pumping really fast and puts you on the threshold of producing lactic acid. For these reasons, anaerobic exercise is very intense and hard to sustain for more than a minute or two at a time.

When used sparingly and in conjunction with long, slow distance running, anaerobic exercise has been shown to improve one's speed and overall aerobic endurance—i.e., the ability to run longer at varying intensities—which is why so many elite and advanced runners utilize it in their training. In chapter 5, I talked specifically about strength training, which is the very best form of anaerobic exercise. In this chapter, I'm going to focus on high-intensity interval training (i.e., speedwork, repetition training) and other forms of cross-training, such as yoga and Pilates, which have both anaerobic and aerobic elements to them.

To go from a 9-minute mile to an 8-minute mile, you have to train anaerobically as well as aerobically, hitting all three levels of the exercise spectrum: anaerobic, anaerobic/aerobic, and aerobic. The following workouts fall more in the middle of the spectrum, and can be instrumental in helping you shave those last 5 to 15 minutes off your marathon or half-marathon time.

Intervals and VO$_2$ Max

Intervals have been used by elite athletes since the early 1900s as a way to stimulate the heart and optimize performance. The theory is that by alternating short periods of high-intensity exercise (at or close to anaerobic state) with slower, less-intense activity (i.e., rest intervals), athletes will improve their maximal oxygen consumption, or VO$_2$ max, and their cardiovascular endurance. The higher your VO$_2$ max, the more efficiently your body utilizes oxygen and the longer it's able to endure under strenuous activity. For example, if you increase your VO$_2$ max, that quarter-mile hill you used to dread so much will feel relatively easy, whereas if your VO$_2$ max remains low, you'll get winded fairly quickly. It's like getting better fuel economy in your car. Many elite distance runners incorporate intervals into their training because this has been shown to improve their aerobic performance over a longer period of time, and make marathon pace feel easier.

Should everyone do interval training? For novice runners who are training for their very first race, it's probably not the wisest idea. They simply don't have the mileage under their belts or the strength and endurance to withstand the rigors of interval training. They'd be best served running a lot of long, slow distances and getting themselves used to being on their feet for several hours. But for the intermediate and advanced runner whose primary goal is to run faster, interval training can definitely mean the difference between a 4:05 and a 3:55 finish in a marathon.

A big misconception about intervals is that they have to be designed to bring you to your knees—a super-high-intensity workout defined by pain and lactic acid building up in your legs. But the reality is that any run pace faster than lactate threshold (when lactic acid starts to accumulate in the blood) can be classified as high intensity. For the intermediate runner, this may amount to anything faster than marathon pace. For the advanced runner, it may be slightly faster than half-marathon pace or even 10K pace.

One goal of running intervals, besides increasing your VO_2 max, is to learn pace separation, says Matthew Moran, PhD, director of the Undergraduate Exercise Science program at Sacred Heart University in Fairfield, Connecticut. This way, you understand the difference between your training pace and your marathon pace, half-marathon pace, and so on.

"Training at different intensities not only will elicit an improved physiological effect, but it is also much more interesting for the runner," Moran says. "The monotony of marathon training at the same pace throughout is unbearable, so the inclusion of different paces is important. I'll have my athletes do a lot of intervals at half-marathon, marathon, and 10K pace, so they know what these paces are in terms of their intervals. This makes it a lot easier for them because they don't have to worry about percentages of intensity. They're just thinking in terms of what they'd do for a 10K race."

One problem, however, with most recreational runners today is that they're fixated on their split times. As a result, they spend too much time training at their lactate threshold (i.e., running too fast), and they're not even aware they're doing it. Their normal easy, relaxed training runs are performed at such a high intensity that when it comes time to run faster, they can't. They've already maxed out.

High-intensity training can be a very effective variable in terms of boosting performance, but only when it's used sparingly.

"The principle of progression should apply to the percentage of training intensity, just as it does to weekly training volume," says Moran, whose RUNtrix algorithms power the customized 12- and 16-week official training programs for the New York City Marathon and NYC Half. "So novice runners should try to understand their paces and start training at intensities that are not too high, and then introduce higher-intensity running into the mix via tempo, fartlek [in which the pace is varied frequently during the run], or interval sessions. It really needs to go in this order. If they try to introduce more intense running first without making sure the majority of their runs are at the correct [lower-intensity] pace, they may end up with a 50-50 split of intensity. And that's trouble. Training doesn't need to feel hard every day. If it does, then something is wrong."

Just what percentage of your training should include these higher-intensity runs? The general rule of thumb—and the one followed by most elite athletes—is that 80 percent or more of your training runs should be maintenance runs, or low-intensity workouts, and 20 percent or less be intervals. Each maintenance run should stimulate your aerobic system, and will typically require you to run at about 65 to 72 percent of your VO_2 max, Moran says. Your higher-intensity workouts should be any run pace faster than lactate threshold, which, according to a 2009 Norwegian study on interval and endurance training, occurs at about 87 percent of your VO_2 max and 90 percent of your max heart rate. You can determine your max heart rate by subtracting your age from 220. Some well-trained athletes can run at 88 percent of max intensity, which puts them right at the cusp of lactate production. The more often they find themselves at or close to this threshold point, the easier it becomes to recognize it and maintain their intensity at that pace.

Here are two interval workouts designed by Moran that you can include in your training. They are both creative and intense, without being intimidating or dangerous for those runners who are new to speedwork. While I don't recommend interval training for beginners or less experienced runners, if you insist on trying it, make sure to start slowly and get accustomed to the different paces before introducing intervals into the mix. Consider running in a few races (5K and 10Ks, 4- and 5-milers, etc.) to help acclimate yourself to these different paces. And once you start doing speedwork, limit yourself to no more than one interval session per week.

Marathon-Pace Repeats

✤ Start with at least a 1-mile warm-up at an easy, relaxed pace and then run 1,000 meters (.625 miles on your GPS watch, or 2½ laps on a quarter-mile track) at your race pace (6:52 per mile for a 3-hour marathon; 9:09 for 4 hours; 11:27 for 5 hours, etc.). Slow down to a very relaxed, easy pace for approximately 30 seconds, and then repeat the 1,000 meters at race pace. Keep repeating the workout to fit your needs and current level of conditioning. It may be that you can do only 2 or 3 repeats the first time around. The goal is to progress to 10 1,000-meter repeats, or 6.2 miles total. You might introduce a few hills into your intervals to make them more challenging, but the key is to keep the rest intervals fairly tight (no more than 75 seconds) in between each repeat.

If you're relatively new to this type of workout and you find 1,000 meters too daunting, then shorten the distance of the repeats to 800 meters at race pace, but keep the rest intervals tight. It's not a ton of recovery time, but it's enough to break up the monotony of running at race pace for several miles. The more time you spend running at your marathon pace, the more you'll get to know that pace, and the more efficient, or economical, you'll become at that pace.

As you progress and start to run more and more intervals, you might find yourself running slightly faster than your pace time. If this is you, then run every other interval at a bit faster than race pace (or, if you're training for a full marathon, run every other at your half-marathon pace), again keeping the recovery periods short so that your body is fatigued.

Marathon Bookends

✤ This is a slightly more advanced workout that should be saved for later on in your training, after you've run a significant number of marathon-pace repeats. The staple of this workout are the 1-mile marathon-pace repeats you run at the beginning and end of the session—thus the workout's name. After a sufficient warm-up, start with a 1-mile interval at marathon pace (say, 8:30), which should come easy for you at this stage. But here comes the twist: You get only half the normal recovery time before you start your next 1-mile interval, which you'll run at a slightly faster half-marathon pace (e.g., 8:15 pace). From here, each mile repeat should get incrementally faster, perhaps getting down to 10K race pace (8:00) or even faster. Once you get down to 10K pace, you should start to accumulate some lactic acid, at which point your rest intervals should increase to allow for more recovery time. Once you're sufficiently fatigued, you're going to take a shorter rest period again before running your last mile repeat at marathon pace (8:30).

The idea behind this interval workout is to get your body both psychologically and physically prepared to run at your marathon race pace, even when your legs are fatigued. This workout helps simulate the challenging final 10 kilometers of a marathon, when your legs are dead tired and you're doing your best to maintain and manage your pace.

Mid-Run Pickups

✤ Acclaimed running coach Tom Fleming believes that building up volume, or on-your-feet time, is what makes you faster, because the more you run, the stronger and more fit you become aerobically, and the easier it is to run at a sustained pace. He does, however, encourage his athletes to occasionally pick up the pace for 2 to 4 miles in the middle of a longer run—say a 7- or 8-mile run—something he did with regularity back in his training days. The short-distance pickups at race pace introduce a little speed and tempo into your longer runs, which helps increase leg turnover and speed in your distance runs without all the stress on the body that speedwork on a track can create. You also learn to recognize the difference between marathon or half-marathon pace and your normal easy, relaxed pace. It's a fun way to gauge your progress in training and, in many instances, helps develop confidence in runners who find that the pace is fairly easy to sustain for 2 to 3 miles. It lets them know that they can, with more training, reach their goal of running 13.1 or 26.2 miles at their goal pace.

In both the Advanced and Intermediate Marathon Training Programs in chapter 13, you'll see that we've incorporated a mid-long run in each of the 10-day phases. This is the perfect time to run these pickups, as these mid-long runs typically range from about 7 to 10 miles. If you're running 9 miles, warm up by running the first 3 miles at an easy, relaxed pace, then run the next 3 at your marathon or half-marathon race pace before cooling down with a slower, more relaxed 3 miles. If, for example, your goal is to run at an 8-minute pace in the marathon (3:30), you'll want to run the first 3 miles at a relaxed, easy pace (approximately 8:30 to 8:45) and then do a 3-mile pickup at an 8-minute pace before throttling it back down to the relaxed, easy pace for the last 3 miles. Try to incorporate at least one pickup per phase (for advanced runners) or every other phase (intermediate runners).

THE HEART OF THE MATTER

Dr. James Kinderknecht, a specialist in primary care sports medicine at the Hospital for Special Surgery in New York, recommends that if you're going to train with a GPS watch, you find one with a heart rate monitor. Forgoing time and using your heart rate as a barometer is a more effective way to increase VO_2 max, says Kinderknecht, a former team physician at the University of Missouri.

"I think if you want to go faster, you're going to have to use your heart rate," Kinderknecht says. "A lot of soccer programs now have their athletes train with heart monitors, where they want to keep their heart rates in certain zones."

Your maximum heart rate is based on your age. The most popular formula to calculate max heart rate is 220 minus your age; therefore, if you're 45 years old, your max heart rate would be 175. This formula has a standard deviation of plus or minus 0 to 12 beats per minute (bpm), but it's a good place to start. On a typical training run, you want to run at approximately 70 percent of your max heart rate (122 bpm for a 45-year-old) and keep it under 80 percent, Kinderknecht says. Stay in this training zone and you should be able to maintain a relaxed, easy pace and build up your aerobic endurance. To train anaerobically, you'll want your intervals to be at least 80 percent of your max heart rate and push 90 percent or more, he says. The longer you're able to train in this 80 to 100 percent, high-intensity zone, the more you'll increase your VO_2 max.

The advantage to having a high VO_2 max is that it makes it easier for your muscles to extract oxygen from the blood during exercise, thus increasing your aerobic endurance and speed. It also strengthens your heart and lungs and boosts your metabolism, allowing you to recruit more muscle fibers when your body is fatigued. It's also known to improve blood pressure.

Treadmill Push (Motor Off)

✤ Most treadmills have some type of interval workout programmed in, but if you really want to get a heart-pumping workout from this machine, turn off the motor and push the belt yourself, says Kai Fusser, MS, an author, coach, and certified personal trainer based in Orlando, Florida. This way you set the pace—you're not just along for the ride.

Some treadmills are easier to push than others, so find one that offers a minimal amount of resistance, says Fusser, who holds a master's degree in nautical engineering from the University of Oldenburg in Germany. Start by walking for 20 to 30 seconds, leaning slightly forward into the machine as if you were pushing a shopping cart or stroller up a hill. Hold on to the handrail as you push the belt back. Then sprint for 5 to 10 seconds—depending on the level of resistance from the machine and your conditioning. On a scale of 1 to 10, your effort on the sprints should be a 10—you are giving it your all! Slow back down to a walking pace for 30 seconds, and then repeat. Do not get off the machine. Try to do six of these cycles (30 seconds slow "walking" pace, 10 seconds sprinting), for a total of 4 minutes. As your fitness level increases, build up to six cycles at a 1:1 ratio (20 seconds walking pace, 20 seconds sprinting).

Adding the resistance of the belt places a higher demand on the muscles and forces them to work harder to sustain your pace. This form of high-intensity interval training also benefits you by working both your aerobic and anaerobic systems, without placing a high degree of stress on your joints because of the soft, cushioning surface. You'll not only strengthen the major muscles in your legs and core but also increase strength in your connective tissue, which helps you to run faster with less effort. Plus, you'll burn a ton of calories in a short period of time.

You can also vary your workouts on the "motor-free" treadmill by pushing on the belt at different angles. Try walking forward for 30 seconds and then sideways for 10 seconds, repeating each cycle six times for 4 minutes. Pushing at different angles helps strengthen your ankles, knees, glutes, hip abductors, and adductors, plus all the connective tissue. Concentrate on pushing with your glutes, not your quadriceps.

Treadmill Side Shuffle

✤ Turn the motor on so the treadmill is moving at a very low rate of speed (2 to 3 miles per hour). Warm up by walking straight ahead for 1 to 2 minutes, and then turn to your left so that your body is perpendicular to the machine. If the treadmill has side rails, hold on to them gently; otherwise, grab the front rail with your right hand to help with your balance. Shuffle sideways on low speed for about 10 to 20 seconds to work your inner (hip adductors) and outer (hip abductors) thigh muscles, then turn back to face the front of the machine and repeat on the other side. Continue to alternate at a 1:1 ratio between walking forward and shuffling sideways. You can add a level of difficulty by increasing the incline on the machine or by crossing one leg over the other as you hop on your feet from side to side. In the beginning, make sure to hang on to at least one rail for balance. Once you become more efficient at the movement, you can keep your arms and hands at your sides. The hip abductors' most important function while running is to stabilize the hips, and the stronger they are, the longer you'll be able to endure and sustain your pace.

Yoga Workouts

✤ Most people think of yoga in terms of flexibility alone, but it's really one of the best cross-training exercises you can do as a runner. It forces you to inhale and exhale vigorously, which increases your VO_2 max and your body's ability to utilize oxygen efficiently during exercise. Holding and stabilizing each yoga pose also helps develop greater core strength. With yoga, you get a full-body workout, as well as enhanced flexibility, strength, and endurance. I recommend doing yoga as a stand-alone workout on a rest or recovery day. If, however, you're going to work it into your daily routine, I recommend doing it after your run, while your muscles are still warm.

Here are a few good yoga poses for runners.

> Holding and stabilizing each yoga pose also helps develop greater core strength. With yoga, you get a full-body workout, as well as enhanced flexibility, strength, and endurance.

Child Pose

✤ Kneel on the floor with your knees slightly wider than your hips, toes untucked, and big toes touching. Sink your hips back onto your heels, bringing your forehead toward the floor. Extend your arms alongside your ears, resting your palms and forearms on the floor in front of you.

✤ Completely relax your elbows, and feel as if your spine is lengthening through your torso as you hold the pose for 10 full breaths in and 10 full breaths out. If you experience pain in your knees and feet, rest a blanket or pillow between the back of your thighs and calves. Also, if the pressure on your ankles or knees is too much, place a blanket or towel underneath them for a little extra cushioning. Besides being a very relaxing position, the child's pose helps to lengthen the spine, release the lower back, open up the hips and glutes, and stretch the thighs and ankles. Curling your toes under you can also stretch the plantar fascia, the thick fibrous band of connective tissue on the sole of each foot—which, if overused, can lead to a very painful inflammatory condition known as plantar fasciitis (see chapter 9). If you're too uncomfortable stretching the plantar fascia in the Child's Pose, then sit up straight with your buttocks over your ankles and toes curled under.

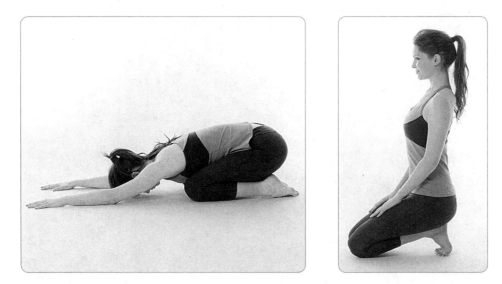

Downward-Facing Dog on Wall

✤ Stand a foot away from a wall and place both hands on the wall at about hip-height, fingers pointing straight up toward the ceiling. With your knees slightly bent, slowly walk your feet away from the wall, until your arms are fully extended and your torso is parallel to the floor. Gradually straighten your legs as far as you can without rounding the back.

✤ Actively push your hands into the wall to lengthen your rib cage and spine. Keep your back flat, and do not allow your shoulder blades to sink toward the floor. Hold this stretch for a count of 10 deep breaths in and out. This exercise really helps to open up your shoulders and chest, while stretching your hips, hamstrings, and calves as well.

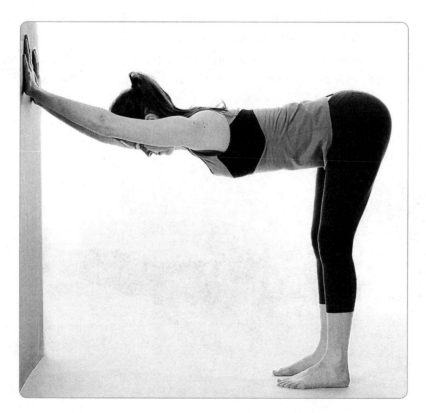

Locust Pose

✣ This is a great full-body pose that helps to open up your chest and strengthen the extensor muscles in your spine, thereby reversing habitual slumping caused by sitting and running. It's also a good abdominal- and core-strengthening exercise. Lie on your stomach with your arms long at your sides, palms facing up. Interlace your fingers or, if you can't make your hands touch, hold a towel behind your back. Press your pelvis down into the floor, then inhale as you slowly lift your upper torso and legs up off the floor, reaching your hands strongly away from your shoulders.

✣ Keep the back of your neck long and soft, so that it forms one continuous line with your spine. At this point, your body should form a very gentle C curve, or half-moon shape. Hold for a count of 7 to 10 deep breaths in and out. You can do a gentler version of this exercise by lifting one leg off the floor at a time and keeping your arms on the floor or by extending your arms out in front of you like Superman and raising the opposite arm and leg together. It doesn't matter how high you raise your legs, as long as they are relatively straight and your knees are off the floor.

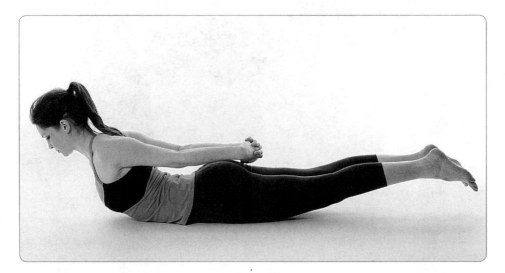

Pilates Workouts

The discipline of Pilates puts an even greater emphasis on the core—the muscles between your rib cage and mid-thighs. A strong, well-functioning core not only stabilizes your pelvis and promotes proper running biomechanics, but also helps transfer power from your arms on down to your feet for more speed. Here are a few Pilates exercises you can do at home that will have a tremendous benefit out on the road.

The Hundred

✤ Lie flat on your back with your knees bent and your arms extended at your sides. Engage your abs by drawing your navel in toward your spine, and then raise one leg at a time into a tabletop position (thighs perpendicular to the floor, shins parallel to the floor). Next, straighten your legs and reach your hands toward your knees, so that your shoulders and then your head come up off the floor. With both arms extended and parallel to the floor, pump your arms up and down for a count of 10 full breaths in and out.

✤ Try to keep a steady rhythm to your arms and your breathing while keeping your head and neck in alignment with your spine. To help ease the pressure on your neck, tuck your chin into your chest and look at your navel while you're performing the movements. If you still feel tension in the neck, then rest your head on a pillow. The ultimate goal is to work up to 100 total pumps (each up-and-down movement counts as 1 pump) for a great abdominal and core workout.

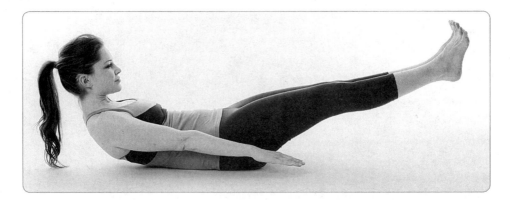

Prone Leg Beats

✛ This exercise will help shape your butt, make your glutes stronger, and also work your hamstrings and lower back muscles. Lie comfortably on your stomach with your heels touching each other, toes pointed back straight, and hands folded underneath your chin or forehead. Rotate your hips underneath you so that your pelvis is in contact with the floor and, with the help of your abdominals, lift both legs and knees together up off the floor. Tap the insides of your heels together, keeping the movement fairly rapid as you inhale and exhale slowly to a count of 10 breaths.

✛ Keep both legs straight and imagine the line between the base of your spine and your neck is lengthening as you tap your heels together.

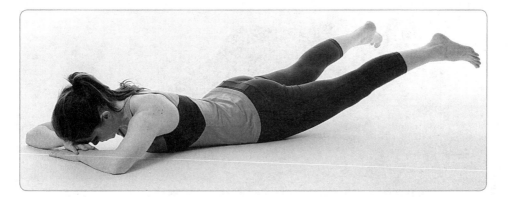

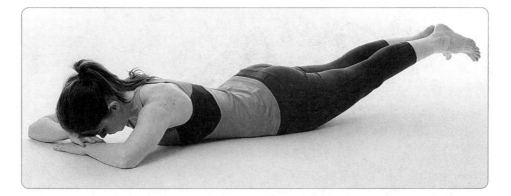

Mountain Climbers

✤ This exercise challenges your core and entire body, and it increases your aerobic endurance without your having to get on a bike, an elliptical machine, or other piece of equipment. Take a position on all fours with your knees, hands, and toes touching the floor. Extend one leg back and lift the other knee off the floor, so that you look like a sprinter in the blocks (you can also start this exercise from a push-up position). Keeping your hands still and butt down, alternately swing the knee of your extended leg forward (toward your hands) in a brisk, jumping fashion, as if you were climbing a mountain. Continue alternating the knees as fast as you can for 30 to 60 seconds, modifying the pace based on your fitness level.

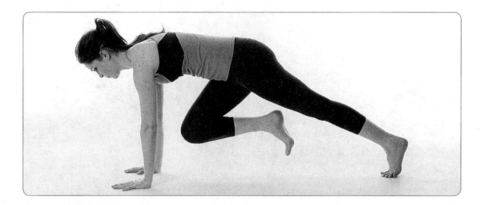

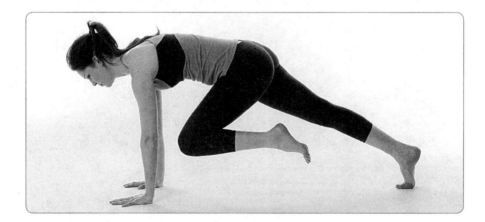

Various Other Forms of Cross-Training

Your local gym (or perhaps even your garage) is full of exercise equipment that you can use to optimize your performance on race day. Of all of these instruments, I like the StairMaster the best, since it's functional (i.e., used in a similar upright fashion to running), low impact, and very good at developing strength in your calves, quads, hamstrings, and glutes—the big guns in running. Make sure not to develop any bad habits like hiking your hips or bending your body to one side when on the Stair-Master. The elliptical machine is also very good for maintaining strength while preserving your joints. Biking is a non-weight-bearing activity, so while it's good for maintaining endurance, it's not going to do much in terms of strengthening your key running muscles. It is, however, one of the best ways to cross-train while you're nursing an injury. Running or walking in the pool is another low-impact exercise that's great for building cardiovascular fitness.

7

Pre- and Post-Run

TO STRETCH OR NOT TO STRETCH? THIS IS ONE OF THE MORE HOTLY debated topics in running, and seemingly everyone has an opinion. Should you stretch before you run, or should you simply lace up your shoes and hit the road?

The most recent science on the subject might make your former gym teacher or youth track and field coach blush. It suggests that static stretching (simply holding a pose for a specific amount of time before you run) has no effect on your performance whatsoever. Moreover, it does little to prevent injury and in some instances even increases the likelihood of your getting hurt.

A clinical trial conducted several years ago and sponsored by USA Track & Field examined more than 2,700 runners and found that those who stretched for 3 months prior to running had similar injury rates to those who didn't stretch at all. Furthermore, those who switched from a non-stretch to a stretch routine for the study increased their injury risk by 22 percent. Another 2013 study conducted by the Department of Kinesiology and Health Science at Stephen F. Austin State University in Texas found that passive static stretching before exercise can actually lead to greater instability and weakness in the stretched musculature. Researchers had several young men (ages 18 to 24) warm up one of two ways prior to performing a barbell squat: statically stretching the lower musculature or dynamically using resistance training equipment. Following static stretching, there was a significant decrease in lower-body stability (22.7 percent) and the amount of weight they could squat (8.3 percent).

It should be noted, however, that many of the studies out there have dealt with weight training and other sports that rely on speed and power, and not endurance activities like running. Also, the test subjects tend to be young, not baby boomers or athletes in their 30s and 40s, which make up the biggest demographic of runners today.

"There's no evidence that supports stretching of any kind, but all of the stretching studies have been done in a population that doesn't need to stretch," says Dr. James Kinderknecht, the primary care sports medicine specialist at New York's Hospital for Special Surgery. "All the data says stretching is not important, but it's shown it's not important in an age group that may not be appropriate to you. This whole concept that stretching before [exercise] is bad—no one has really said that."

Dr. Kinderknecht believes that the most effective way to warm up for a run is dynamically, proceeding from a walk to a very slow-pace jog to running. But because of time restraints, most runners don't want to allocate 5 minutes of their 45-minute run to walking or jogging. They're usually so crunched for time that their warm-up consists of putting on their clothes and jogging down their steps.

"I think you're much better served doing a dynamic workout, such as a nice, brisk 5-minute walk, then progressing into your training run," says Matthew Moran, the Undergraduate Exercise Science program director at Sacred Heart University. "One of the hardest things to do is to get people to start their training runs slow. The Kenyans start running at a grandma-like pace—it's mind-boggling how slow they start. Yet it's because they warm up in such a gradual, linear fashion that they're able to run faster later on."

Still, there remain many advantages to stretching beforehand, especially if the runner is prone to tightness and fatigue. Dr. Joseph Feinberg, the Hospital for Special Surgery's chief physiatrist and the team physician for St. Peter's University, says that as runners age and more degenerative changes occur to their bodies, stretching becomes more important, especially in areas like the calves, Achilles tendons, and iliotibial band, which don't receive much in the way of blood flow.

"The one thing stretching may be good for prior to running is increasing blood flow," Feinberg says. "You need blood flow to muscles and tissues for them to be able to contract efficiently. And then there are the tendons, where a lot of overusage occurs. There are watershed areas in the tendon, and if they're too tight, then the tension decreases blood flow to the tendon. If the tendon has diminished blood flow, it's more likely to get injured."

It's also very important that you strengthen the muscle-tendon junctions and joints in these problem areas, in particular the weight-bearing structures around your feet, ankles, and knees. Most people interpret tightness as "I've got to stretch more," but in many instances that tightness is a product of fatigue. Rather than stretch the muscles, you'd be better served by strengthening them and the supporting structures around them.

There is no absolute rule for stretching, but for most runners—especially those over the age of 40—I highly recommend that you incorporate a dynamic warm-up (walking briskly or jogging slowly at the start) into your routine prior to running. For those of you who prefer to stretch, you're much better off doing a resistive-type form of stretching (dynamic stretching) versus just hanging out in a stretch and holding the point of tension for 30 seconds or more. Dynamic stretching allows you to work slowly to the limits of your full range of motion, and is much more effective in terms of getting the muscle tissue and musculoskeletal system prepared for the loading that goes on during running. Static stretching should be reserved for after your runs, when your body's core temperature is very warm and your muscles are relaxed.

The following pre-run stretches, designed by physical therapist Patricia Ladis, cofounder of KIMA Center for Physiotherapy and Wellness in New York City, add a dynamic element to some common running stretches for your calves, glutes, hamstrings, hip flexors, and other major running-specific muscle groups. This way, you're not simply stretching the muscle fibers but you're also warming them up through a full range of motion using various controlled movements. Hold the dynamic, or resistance, part of each of the movements for 5 seconds before releasing and then repeating again several times. All of these stretches should be performed within 15 minutes of starting your run.

Calf and Achilles Stretch

✣ Stand approximately 2 feet from a wall (or railing) with your hips facing the wall. Place your hands on the wall and then extend your left leg behind you with your heel flat on the ground. Flare your left foot in, using your toes, to open up more of the muscle fibers in your calf. Lean gently into the wall until you start to feel a good stretch in your left calf, and then lift and drop your left heel to the ground.

✣ Repeat 10 times in a continuous lift-and-drop motion to stretch the gastrocnemius, or large bulging calf muscle at the back of your leg. Next, return to the starting position and bend your left knee forward (toward the wall) to work more of the soleus (lower calf muscle responsible for flexing the foot downward) and Achilles tendon (photo, opposite page). You may need to narrow your stance from the one you used for the dynamic stretch above. Keeping the knee bent, lift and lower the heel to the ground as before.

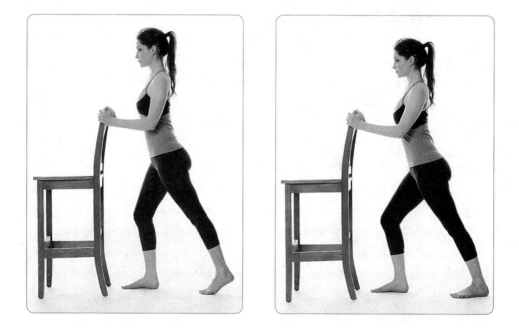

✤ Repeat 9 more times, pumping the heel up and down while keeping the knee bent and pointing straight ahead, over the second toe. Switch legs and repeat to increase the range of motion and blood flow to these vital weight-bearing muscles and tendons, which not only help absorb impact but also allow the feet to extend and flex as you land and push off the ground.

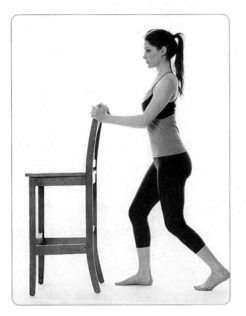 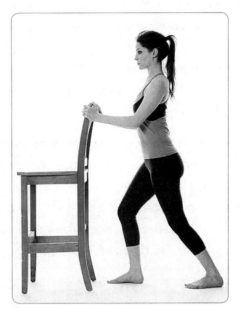

Hamstring Stretch

✤ This stretch targets the hamstrings, which are responsible for both bending (flexion) and extending the knees, as well as extending the hips. As the legs swing forward, the hamstrings are stretched, so it's very important to keep these muscles as pliant and flexible as possible. From a standing position, take a slightly staggered stance, positioning the toes of your left foot up against a wall, high chair, or tree. Your left leg should be extended and your right leg somewhat behind you, bent at the knee. Keeping your left leg straight and your back flat, bow forward and stick your butt out. You should now begin to feel a good stretch in your left hamstring, just above the knee.

✤ To add a dynamic element to the stretch, press down into the floor with your left foot as if you were going to pull it back, then bow forward. Hold for up to 5 seconds, release, and bow forward into the newly gained range of motion or stretch. Repeat again, pushing the left foot down to further contract the hamstring and then relaxing the muscle. Repeat up to 5 more times and then switch legs, remembering to keep your back flat, bowing forward from the creases of your hips.

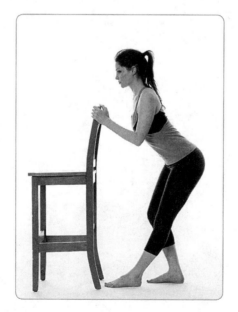

Quad Stretch

✤ This exercise targets the quadriceps muscles at the front of your thigh, a large group of muscles responsible for extending and straightening the legs, as well as flexing the hips. It also plays an important role in stabilizing the knees. From a standing position, reach behind you with your right hand and grab your right foot. You may want to extend your left arm straight out in front of you or hold on to something to help with balance. Next, pull your right foot up toward your right buttocks and bring your right knee in toward your left.

✤ Then, without allowing your right knee to slide forward, press the knee into your standing-leg (left) knee, and tuck your tailbone in underneath you. To make the stretch dynamic, press the top of your right foot down toward the floor as if you were going to extend your right knee, only resist the movement with your right hand. Hold for 5 seconds, release, and then repeat several more times before switching legs. Always try to keep the fronts of your thighs aligned and your knees touching.

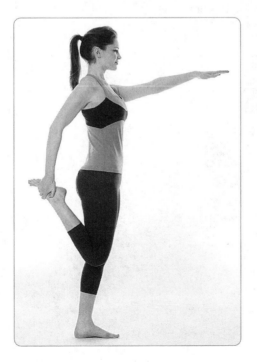

Hip Flexor Stretch

✤ The hip flexors are an important group of muscles in running, as they're responsible for lifting your knees and bringing your hips forward as you run, giving you that fast, powerful leg drive. Unfortunately, if you lead a very sedentary lifestyle, these muscles can sit in a very shortened, weakened state for too long. They need to be warmed up and lengthened dynamically before you run. To stretch the hip flexors dynamically, get in a forward lunge position on the floor with your right leg bent in front of you and your left leg trailing behind you, knee flat on the floor. Apply pressure down into the floor with your right foot, simultaneously pressing through the floor with your left knee as if you were trying to bring that leg forward.

✤ Hold for several seconds, engaging the hip flexors in your upper left thigh, then release and repeat again. Squeezing the glutes will provide an even greater stretch in the hip flexors. If you want to stretch the quads, too, place your trailing foot up on a bench or up against a stationary object, such as the bark of a tree. Repeat the stretch with the left leg in front.

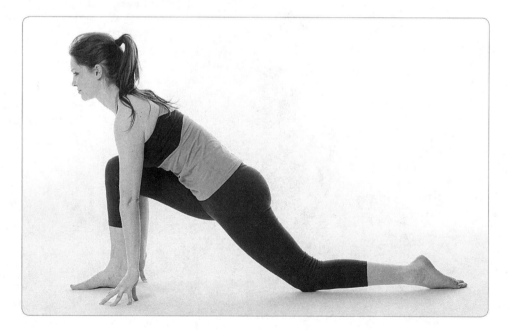

Bowler Exercise (For Hip Abductors)

✤ This exercise improves the strength and functioning of the gluteus medius muscle, the primary hip abductor muscle of the outer thigh, located just behind your hip pocket. It is an important stabilizer of the pelvis and plays a major role in preventing many common running injuries. In particular, it helps to take the load off the iliotibial band and lower back; it also allows you to use your push-off muscles more efficiently. From a standing position, shift your weight onto your left leg and then cross your right leg behind you as if you were dropping down into a position to throw a bowling ball. Your left leg should be soft and slightly bent, and your right leg should simply hang out at about a 45-degree angle. From this position, sink your weight into your standing hip as if you were wagging an imaginary tail to the left. Next, come up into a straight-knee position on your standing leg, pushing up through your left glute so that the hip is more underneath you.

✤ Then repeat again, wagging the imaginary tail to the left as you sink into the hip, then pressing through the glute and lifting the hip. Perform 10 movements on your left leg and then repeat on your right leg.

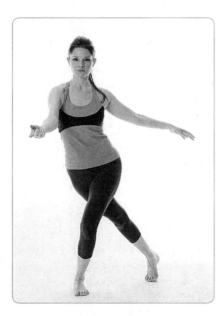 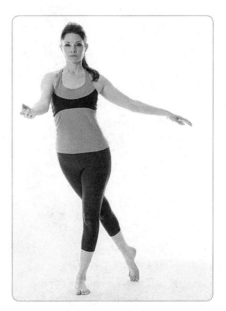

Figure-Four Stretch (For Glutes)

✤ This is a very effective dynamic stretch to warm up the large buttock muscles, or glutes, which are responsible for accelerating the body forward as well as stabilizing the hips. From a standing position, cross your right leg in front of you and rest your right ankle on top of your left knee so that your legs form a figure four. From here, squat down into the hip of your bent (right) leg, until you feel a good stretch in your right glute.

✤ Sit there for a moment, and then push your right ankle down into your left knee. By resisting back, you will engage the gluteus muscles even more, as well as the external hip rotators, enhancing their range of motion and effectiveness. Hold the resistance phase of this stretch for up to 10 seconds, release the pressure, and then repeat again several more times before switching legs.

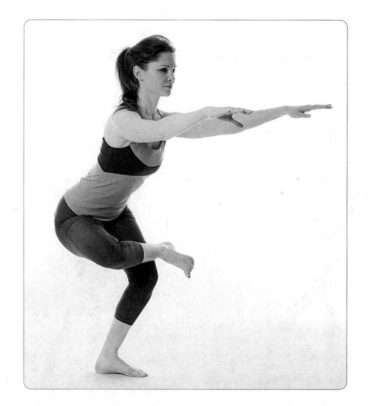

Leg Swings (For Lower Back Pain, Sciatica)

✣ This is a great stretch and release for runners who suffer from lower back pain or sciatic pain deep in the rear and back of the thigh. It flosses the sciatic nerve (meaning you're moving the nerve through a small range of motion to help loosen the connective tissue around the nerve; you pull from one end of the nerve while keeping the other end relaxed, freeing the nerve from any adhesions along the way) as well as other spinal nerves to help relieve some of the pressure and discomfort caused by the compression of these nerves. Stand up straight and then bring your left foot up off the ground so that all of your weight is supported by your right leg. You can also stand with your right foot on a curb and let the left leg dangle. Keeping your spine and pelvis in a very still, neutral position (no bending or swaying back and forth or from side to side), swing your left leg straight forward and back in a pendulum fashion, using only your left hip as a fulcrum.

✣ Look straight ahead as you swing the leg from the hip; looking down can tense the nerve. Complete about 12 swings and then repeat on the other leg, again keeping your entire trunk still as you move freely through the hip of your swinging leg. In addition to releasing pressure on the nerve, it dynamically strengthens the standing leg.

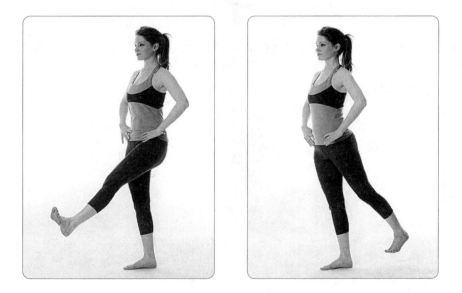

Jumping Body Twists (For Mid-Back Stiffness)

✤ Because many runners sit at a desk 8 hours a day or more, they find themselves with very tight, shortened pelvic muscles and a rigid, stiff back with little thoracic rotation. When you get little movement from your mid- and upper back, you place greater loads on your lumbar spine and lower back, putting you at a higher risk for injury. To open up the thorax region, between your head and abdomen, try the following dynamic stretch prior to running. From a standing position, raise your arms to chest height and stick your elbows out as if you were going to perform the funky chicken dance. Both elbows should be pointing away from your sides. Hop up and down on your feet, twisting your hips in one direction while rotating through your mid-back in the other direction.

✤ In other words, as your pelvis twists to the right, your arms and thoracic spine (upper/mid-back) should twist to the left. In addition to increasing your thorax rotation, you'll also get a good, heart-pumping warm-up that also mimics the same activity as running.

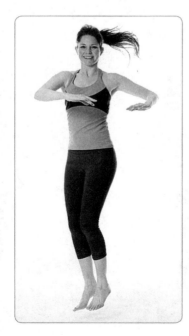

Post-Run Stretches

You'll get very few people to argue about the importance of stretching post-run. The most effective time to stretch is after you run, when the muscles are warm. You create a better stretch, which helps maintain flexibility, strength, and endurance and speeds up recovery. The following stretches should be done within 15 minutes after your run, and in a seated or lying-down position—with the exception of the Standing Side Extensions. The prone and supine positions will assist you in giving each muscle a more targeted stretch. You'll also enjoy being off your feet.

> The most effective time to stretch is after you run, which helps to maintain flexibility, strength, and endurance, and speeds recovery.

Hamstring Stretch

✣ Lie on your back with your right knee bent, left leg extended out in front of you on the floor, and arms at your sides. Bring your right leg up toward you and clasp your hands behind your right thigh (you can use a towel if this is too difficult). Pull the leg toward your chest until you start to feel a good stretch in your right hamstring. Keep your left leg straight and the left knee down as you pull the right leg toward you.

✣ Hold the stretch for 10 deep breaths in and out, and repeat twice more before switching legs. To activate the hamstring even more and stretch it dynamically, push your right leg away from your body into your hands as if you were trying to kick it toward the floor. Resist the movement with your hands, and hold for up to 5 seconds. Release the pressure and take up the slack by pulling the leg closer to you, then repeat this push-pull interval several more times to further increase the range of motion in the hamstring. Switch legs and repeat.

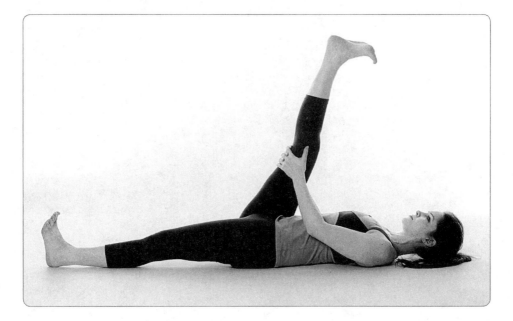

Lying Quad Stretch

✣ Lie on your right side with your right forearm and elbow supporting your body and your left arm at your side. Reach down with your left hand and pull your left foot up toward your buttocks.

✣ See if you can get your left heel to touch your left glute; if you can't, gradually work up to that point. While holding the stretch, make sure that both thighs are parallel to each other and your front side forms a long, straight line from your foot to your resting elbow. Hold for a count of 10 deep breaths in and out, and switch sides to give your quadriceps muscles a good stretch. This group of four muscles at the front of your thigh helps stabilize the knee, as well as bend and control the leg at the hip joint.

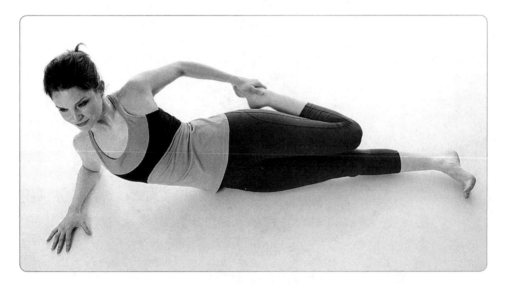

Bound-Angle Seated Stretch

✤ Stretching the groin area will help prevent painful groin strains, which can severely limit your ability to lift your knees and stride efficiently. Take a seat on the ground or floor with your knees bent and the soles of your feet touching. Grab hold of both ankles and lean forward, up away from your hips. Try to keep your spine long and your back as straight as possible.

✤ You can apply gentle pressure to the center of your inner thighs to increase the stretch in your inner thigh area (groin and hip adductor muscles), but be careful not to overuse your arms. Hold for 10 deep breaths in and out and repeat once more.

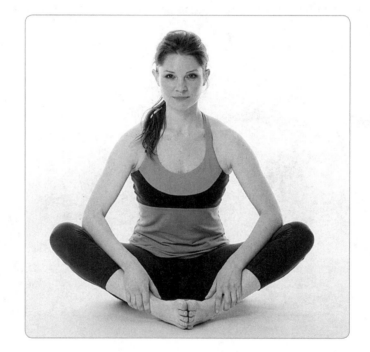

Hip Internal Rotation Stretch

✤ This exercise helps increase the internal rotation of your hips, thus helping stabilize the pelvis. Lie on your back with your knees bent and arms extended out away from your body. Cross your right leg over your left so that the outside of your right ankle rests on the outer part of your left thigh. Then, using the weight of your right leg, pull your left leg to the right and down toward the floor.

✤ To increase the pressure on your left leg, pull your right leg down with your right hand. Hold this position for a count of 10 deep breaths in and out, then return to the starting position and repeat on the other leg. You should feel a good stretch across your thigh and hip.

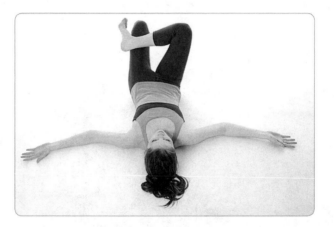

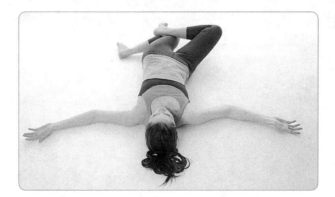

Piriformis Stretch

✤ This exercise stretches the piriformis muscle, which is located deep in the buttocks and is primarily responsible for rotating the thigh laterally. A tight piriformis is often associated with a condition known as piriformis syndrome, in which the sciatic nerve (which passes through the muscle) becomes irritated by the piriformis, causing pain in the buttocks or lower back region. Lie flat on your back with both knees bent and feet flat on the floor. Cross your right leg in front of your left so that the outside of your right ankle rests against the knee. From here, grasp the underside of your left thigh, just below the knee, and pull it gently toward your chest until you feel a stretch in your right glute and hip.

✤ Hold for at least 10 deep breaths in and out, and repeat with the other leg.

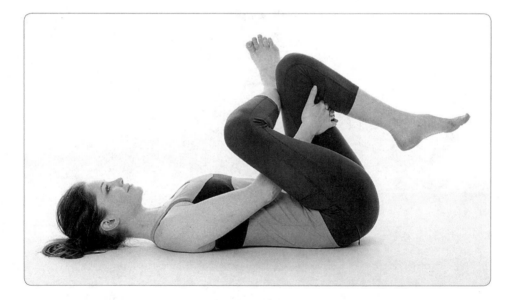

Book Opening

✣ This exercise helps open up the thoracic spine, creating more rotational mobility through your rib cage. It also stretches your chest muscles (pec major and minor), which can get very tight while you're sleeping or after sitting at a desk all day. Lie on your right side with your knees bent up to hip level (90 degrees or so), similar to a fetal position. Extend both arms out in front of you so that both arms are in line with your shoulders. Without moving your lower lumbar spine or your pelvis, reach your top arm up and over your body, rotating your upper body slowly to the left as far as you can. Your head should follow your hands comfortably. Hold for a count of three deep breaths in and out, then slowly return to the starting position and repeat 4 more times before switching onto your left side. Rotate only through your thoracic spine and rib cage, and keep your lower spine, pelvis, and legs completely still.

✣ As you gain flexibility, aim to get your shoulder blades and full arms resting on the floor.

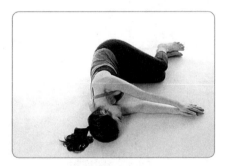 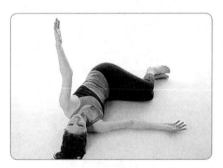

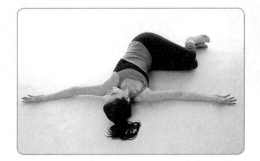

Standing Side Bends/Extensions

✤ Anytime you're stretching the side of your body, you want to lengthen the side you're stretching as tall as possible before you go into a side bend, says Patricia Ladis of KIMA Center for Physiotherapy and Wellness. Stand up straight and extend your left arm straight up toward the sky, reaching up as high as you can (which lengthens the side of your body) as you bend to the right.

✤ Breathe in so that your ribs are extending outward as you reach up toward the sky. Don't let the hips go; focus more on the up (i.e., vertical stretch) instead of the over. You want to lift up out of your standing position and really open up the rib cage before bending slightly to the side, or as far as your range of motion will allow. Hold for about 10 seconds, and then repeat on the other side to open up your obliques, lats, and supporting spinal muscles (paraspinals). This will improve your posture so that you feel nice and long, not short and compressed, as you stride, which in turn will improve your running efficiency and economy.

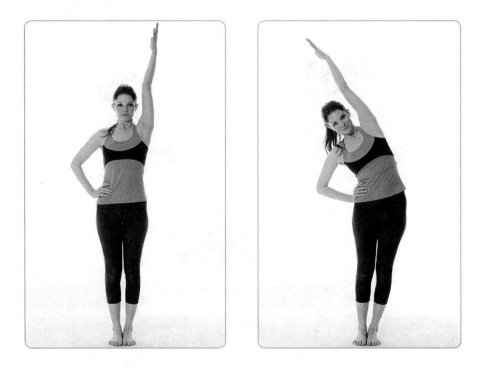

Injury Prevention
and Recovery

A EUROPEAN GENTLEMAN I KNOW ARRIVED IN NEW YORK CITY IN late October 2011 to run in the New York City Marathon. Until the moment I first saw him, he had done almost everything right. In relatively good shape for someone in his early 50s, he had arrived 10 days early to get acclimated to the different time zone and was well hydrated. He seemed good to go, except he panicked. He had apparently missed a week or two of training in the weeks leading up to the race, and, like so many runners in his shoes, he tried to catch up the week prior to the marathon. Instead of taking it easy and continuing to taper, he decided to get in a few more long runs. On consecutive days, he ran 17 and 18 miles in Central Park.

Four days prior to the marathon, he came to see me, complaining of pain in his lower leg. By then, it was too late. He had a stress fracture of the tibia, which generally takes 3 to 6 months to recover from. His marathon was over before it started.

Every October, I see a ton of panicked runners, just like my European friend, with all sorts of overuse injuries. I refer to it as the "October Surprise" because they're always showing up at my office door in late October, just prior to the New York City Marathon. And none of them are 25 years old! Today's average marathoner is getting older (with an average of 39.8 years for men and 36.2 for women), and the older you get, the more time your body needs to recover. You can't run or play basketball every day as you did when you were 20. Running tears up your muscles, and they need to time to repair and rebuild themselves.

It's not always a bone, muscle, or tendon injury, either. One patient of mine, 44-year-old Dan, knew something was wrong about a month before the marathon. The weather had turned a bit cooler in New York, and he found himself breathing more shallowly and rapidly than he ever had before. Dan started laboring through many of his training runs, even the shorter 5-milers, and exhibited some of the classic signs of overtraining, including fatigue, heavy legs, and muscle soreness. But because he was so deep into his training, and the marathon was just around the corner, he felt the need to keep pushing on. He wasn't about to back off. On his last long run, Dan decided to run 20 miles at his goal marathon pace (slightly more than 9 minutes per mile). He thought that knowing he could sustain the desired pace for 20 miles would give him the confidence to break 4 hours on race day. Dan managed to run the 20 miles—which included a half-marathon race—with few hiccups, averaging a 9:04 mile, but the stress of running so hard for so long was more than his body could handle.

Dan came to see me a week prior to the 2012 New York City Marathon complaining of pain on the right side of his rib cage. He couldn't sleep on either side of his body or lie down, and it hurt him to take deep breaths; it felt as if he had broken his ribs. It turned out that he had a case of pleurisy, or pleuritis, an inflammation of the lining of the lungs often brought on by a viral infection. Even if the race had not been canceled in the aftermath of Hurricane Sandy, he still wouldn't have been able to run because of his condition.

In this instance, the viral infection was likely brought on by overtraining. Dan would've been much better off resting or going to see a doctor the minute he recognized something was wrong. At the very least, he should've scaled back his final long run and run it at a normal (relaxed, easy) training pace. But like so many runners, he feared being underprepared on race day and felt the need to get in one more hard long run. He was penny-wise and pound-foolish, and as a result paid the price later on.

Runners are the worst when it comes to listening to their bodies, and unfortunately, that is why so few of them make it to the starting line completely healthy. What's more, runners always think they have to do more, not less, during the latter stages of training. The two examples above clearly show what can happen when you ignore the warning signs of overtraining and don't give your body enough time to recover.

Rule number 1 in the "New Rules of Injury Prevention" is that you're better off resting too much than not resting enough. You need to train and learn to endure, but if missing one long run is necessary to get your body 100 percent ready for race day, then you're much better off skipping that run.

Here are several other injury prevention rules you should consider:

Increase Your Mileage Gradually

As a general rule of thumb, try not to increase your mileage by more than 10 percent over the previous week, or 10-day phase—as it's known in our full-marathon training programs. This means that if you run 25 miles in the first phase, keep it to about 28 miles in the next one. Our programs are designed to get you to run more, but in a very gradual, progressive fashion. If you're consistent in this manner and you don't increase your mileage too rapidly, you'll stand a good chance of getting to the starting line of your race healthy.

Alternate Hard and Easy Days

Every time you run, you deplete your body's energy stores and damage your muscles and connective tissues. They need time to replenish and repair themselves, and when you're training more than you're resting, you're very likely to become a victim of an overtraining injury. "Most running injuries are the result of inadequate rest or recovery time," says CUNY York College clinician and health science professor Dr. Shawn Williams. "Rest is the most important, efficient recovery workout there is. When you're resting, your parasympathetic nervous system starts to kick in, and metabolism is increased. This accelerates your recovery."

Understand the Symptoms of Overtraining

There are as many as seven established signs of overtraining, and the more you familiarize yourself with them, the better your chance of preventing an irreversible injury that could sideline you for a big race. The most obvious of these signs is fatigue, or exhaustion—you simply don't have the energy to get out of bed or complete your runs. Part of the reason you may be so tired is that you're not getting enough quality uninterrupted sleep—especially if you're very restless and find yourself waking up a lot in the middle of the night. Interrupted sleep interferes with your body's ability to release endorphins and growth hormones, which help stimulate repair and your body's ability to recover.

Other symptoms of overtraining include depression, frequent colds or illness, crankiness, heavy legs, and muscle soreness that lasts for days. Williams says that many overtrained runners often put aside normal things they do every day outside of running. They frequently show up late to work and also tend to pay less attention to their hygiene habits. Other indicators that you may be overtraining include an elevated resting heart rate in the morning and cloudy, foul-smelling urine. If you start to notice any of these symptoms, give yourself a few days off and see whether they start to go away. If not, then go see your doctor.

Stay Well Hydrated

After muscle overuse, dehydration is the leading cause of injuries in runners. Your body needs to take in more fluids during training to maintain the contraction and relaxation of the muscles. When you become dehydrated, this mechanism is altered, often leading to muscle strains (especially in the hamstrings and calves) and cramps. Depletion of electrolytes, particularly sodium, can also cause muscles to cramp. Electrolytes are responsible for transmitting electrical signals in the body so that your muscles continue to fire as you run.

Follow a Diet Rich in Anti-inflammatory Foods

One of the things that happens to your body after the age of 40 is that your tissues begin to lose water—about 1 percent each year. Your muscles, ligaments, tendons, and cartilage have a harder time retaining water, which, among other things, contributes to a lack of flexibility and strength. Your discs may also start to show signs of wear and tear and lose their ability to act as shock absorbers. Water loss is one of the biggest contributors to degenerative disc disease.

Don't confuse this water loss with dehydration, however—you can't drink your way out of aging. But what you can do to protect these tissues is exercise regularly and follow a healthy diet rich in vitamins, antioxidants, and omega-3s. These anti-inflammatory foods will help you maintain a healthy weight, thus reducing the loads on your musculoskeletal system. They also promote a faster healing process. Stay away from processed foods and beverages rich in high-fructose corn syrup, such as candy, soda, and baked goods. This sweetener increases inflammation in the body and is also known to raise your resistance to insulin, promoting more weight gain. Make sure your diet consists of berries, fruits, vegetables, nuts, whole grains, fish, and other anti-inflammatory foods shown to reduce your resistance to insulin.

Consider Hormone Optimization Therapy

As we age, our levels of hormones (estrogen in women, testosterone in men) start to diminish. This condition, known as menopause in women and andropause—or male menopause—in men, typically occurs in one's 40s or 50s. For women, menopause marks the end of their monthly period cycle and reproductive stage. Menopause occurs at a much more rapid pace than andropause and is also known to dramatically speed up bone loss as well. Estrogen is an anabolic hormone that helps increase bone density, and after menopause the ovaries stop producing this hormone. As a result, postmenopausal women are at a much greater risk of sustaining bone fractures and, later in life, osteoporosis. While andropause occurs at a much slower rate, it is often accompanied by a lower-than-normal sex drive and feelings of lethargy. Testosterone helps stimulate muscle growth, and once this stimuli begins to fade, you start to lose muscle, vigor, and energy.

As your hormone levels start to decline, your risk of getting osteoporosis or suffering an injury to your bones, muscle-tendon junctions, and cartilage increases—especially if you're not giving your body enough time to rest and recover. In recent years, anti-aging and hormone replacement supplements have become big business in the multibillion-dollar supplement industry. You see as many commercials on television today touting these anti-aging hormone supplements as you do peddling sexual enhancement pills. Provided it's supervised and the benefits outweigh the risks, small-dose testosterone or estrogen replacement therapy can help relieve symptoms associated with the decline of both hormones. It has been shown to help minimize muscle and bone loss with aging. But this type of therapy has risks, especially if you continue it after the age of 70. Men at this age are at a greater risk for developing testicular or liver cancer, whereas women have an increased risk of heart disease or breast or uterus cancer. You should consult your doctor before beginning any hormone optimization therapy, and if your family has a history of heart disease or any of the cancers mentioned above, you should probably steer clear of it.

Other, less risky supplements you may want to consider include 1-TetraDecanol Complex (1-TDC), an extremely powerful natural anti-inflammatory and advanced form of fatty acid that suppresses the negative aspects of inflammation without interrupting the natural healing process, curcumin (for cartilage), fish oil (a natural anti-inflammatory), and vitamin D. Active runners, especially women, should get their vitamin D levels tested annually to make sure they don't have a deficiency in this all-important vitamin, which helps in the absorption of calcium and in maintaining strong bone health.

I should warn you that some recent studies have linked fish oil supplements to an increased risk of prostate cancer in men; however, it's also been shown to reduce the risk of breast cancer in women.

Manage Your Thyroid

If you suffer from fatigue, abnormal weight gain, depression, baldness, or sensitivity to cold, it could be not that you're overtraining but rather that you have an underactive thyroid gland. This means that the thyroid is not producing enough of the hormones triiodothyronine and thyroxine. These two hormones help regulate your body's metabolism and energy use. You can take supplements to help replace these lost hormones, much as you can to help with the effects of menopause and andropause, but without the same risks as with estrogen and testosterone supplementation. If left untreated, an underactive thyroid can lead to kidney failure, heart disease, and early menopause in women. It can also negatively affect blood flow and lead to more wear on cartilage and tendons as well. An underactive thyroid is generally not considered very serious, but it is recommended that you have these hormone levels checked (through a simple blood test) every year after age 40.

Hit the Weights

Yet another reason to wish you were 25 again is that as you get older, the muscle-tendon junctions in the body receive even less blood flow, particularly in the inner core of the tendons. As a result, areas with already decreased blood circulation, like the Achilles tendon, calf muscles, and hamstrings, become even more susceptible to injury.

One way to keep these weight-bearing tendons, ligaments, and bones healthy is to strength-train several times per week. This helps minimize muscle and bone loss, especially in women. Strength training increases bone density by aiding in the remodeling, or rebuilding, of the bones, thus reducing the risk of osteoporosis and stress fractures. Stronger muscles also help to stabilize your body and can handle greater workloads, or distances such as 26.2 miles.

Avoid the Sidewalk

Whenever possible, avoid concrete and stick to softer surfaces such as dirt, cinder, firm sand, or, if you have to run on the road, asphalt. The softer the surface, the better it is for your joints and long-term health. Hard concrete surfaces, such as sidewalks, can really deliver a shock to your joints and cause shin splints if you're not used to running on them. You can also minimize overuse injuries by avoiding heavily slanted or cambered roads and running on the flattest part of the road, and by alternating the direction in which you run. If you consistently run in the same direction, then you increase the risk of injury—such as meniscal or labral tears—in your downhill leg.

BIOCHEMICAL CONSIDERATIONS FOR RUNNERS

Bright-colored fruits and vegetables are rich in antioxidants, which inhibit the oxidation of other molecules and help prevent cellular damage that can be caused by free radicals. Eat these often! As a runner, you face greater demands on your cells and therefore produce more of these unstable free radicals, which, under high oxidative stress, can damage tissue and accelerate the progression of cancer, cardiovascular disease, and age-related diseases such as Alzheimer's and Parkinson's.

Your best defense against these free radicals is (1) to not overtrain and (2) to overload on antioxidants. Good sources of antioxidants include foods rich in vitamins C and E and beta-carotene, such as berries, apples, beans, nuts, chocolate, and coffee. Fruit juices, particularly pomegranate and berry juices, are also excellent choices. You should avoid smoking and drinking too much alcohol while training, as they, too, can increase oxidative stresses on the cells.

Dr. Shawn Williams, who has subspecialty certifications with USA Track & Field, recommends that you also get tested for the following biochemical markers, all of which can undergo changes when the body is placed under stress (such as from running or other exercise). Most of these can be checked with a simple blood test:

1. Vitamin B: B vitamins help your cells make energy and protect your nerves and help regulate inflammation.
2. Amino acids: These acids are the building blocks for muscle tissue and tissue regeneration. They play a role in virtually every system in the body.

3. Essential fatty acids: Omega-3 and omega-6 fats help to control and regulate a healthy inflammatory response that promotes healing.
4. Magnesium: This mineral is involved in more than 300 reactions in the body, including muscle relaxation, sleep, and energy production.
5. Zinc: This mineral plays an important role in the management of insulin (a growth hormone), testosterone, inflammation, and cardiovascular health.

The Road to a Faster Recovery

Many of the rules of prevention and recovery are intertwined, none more so than the need for rest, or recovery days. As Dr. Williams has said, "Rest is the most important, efficient recovery workout." When your body is at rest, it flushes out the lactic acid it accumulated during your last hard run. It starts to repair micro-tears and other damage that has been done to it, and to rebuild these live tissues so that you're even stronger for your next run.

But the entire process takes time, and if you continue to run hard every day, you won't give your body enough time to heal and regenerate itself. One of the hardest things for runners to do is make themselves take a easy, relaxed run of 5, 6, or 7 miles. They want to run at race pace all the time. Remember: Training is cumulative, and if you train too hard, eventually the fatigue and stress will catch up to you. The key to surviving marathon training is to make sure that the vast majority of your runs are relaxed and easy (i.e., at a conversational pace). You shouldn't be working hard every time you head out the door. Save those efforts for your long runs and faster-tempo workouts. Most studies today show that if you train a body really hard and then give it days to recover, it will come back even stronger and faster. That doesn't mean you have to take 2 days completely off after every hard effort—for some, an easy, relaxed 6-mile run constitutes a recovery day—but if you follow the hard-easy-easy system in all three marathon training programs in chapter 13, you will recover faster and start to see your running efficiency improve.

Here are some rules of recovery for you to keep in mind as you train:

1. Hit the Pillows: Make sure to allow for enough time for rest. While there's no magic number, the National Sleep Foundation recommends that adults get between 7 and 9 hours of sleep every day. And that's for the average adult, not one who's training to run in a marathon or half-marathon.

The only time your body can rebuild itself is when it's at rest. Your body recovers best when it's resting comfortably, so strive to get at least 6 to 8 hours of sleep per day.

2. Stretch It Out: The best time to stretch is immediately after you've run, while your muscles are still warm and in a very elastic state. You'll create a better stretch, improve your overall flexibility, and flush out lactic acid and other toxins from your muscles to help speed recovery and prevent soreness. Refer back to chapter 7 for seven of the very best post-run stretches.

3. Refuel and Rehydrate: As soon as you finish stretching, make sure to give your body the necessary nutrients it needs to rehydrate, repair, and refuel itself so that you can come back even stronger for your next effort. One of the very best post-run drinks to aid in this process is low-fat chocolate milk, because it contains the recommended 3:1 ratio of carbohydrates to protein, as well as electrolytes (sodium). Your body needs the carbs to replenish the energy (glycogen stores) it lost during the run, and the protein to assist in repairing damaged muscle tissues. The sooner you consume one of these drinks after your run, the faster your body can recover.

4. Chill Out: A staple of many elite runners' post-run recovery is the ice bath. The chilly water constricts blood flow to the damaged muscles, thus reducing swelling, inflammation, and tissue breakdown. The cold minimizes your body's inflammatory response to the damaged tissue and other harmful stimuli threatening your body, and initiates the healing process to speed up your recovery. To take an ice bath, fill your tub with cold water from the tap, climb in, and dump in one to two 5-pound bags of ice. For the best results, take your ice bath within an hour of completing your run, preferably after doing a deep-tissue massage with a foam roller (see next page). Stay in the tub for approximately 20 minutes or until the ice melts.

5. Supplement Your Body: While Advil, Aleve, and other over-the-counter pain relievers are okay if taken in moderation, there are some much safer natural anti-inflammatory alternatives to these non-steroidal anti-inflammatory drugs (NSAIDs). Vitamin D, fish oil, and curcumin all help with the recovery of muscles, tendons, and ligaments and have none of the side effects (high blood pressure, bleeding ulcers, kidney damage) associated with NSAIDs (although, as noted, some recent studies have linked fish oil to an increased risk of prostate cancer in men). Vitamin D also promotes good bone health. The recommended daily dosage for each is as follows: vitamin D: 1,000 units; fish oil: 2,000 milligrams; curcumin: 1,500 milligrams.

GOOD DAILY VITAMINS AND SUPPLEMENTS

- 1-TetraDecanol Complex (1-TDC): Take 3 soft gel tablets of this unique fatty acid daily (orally); apply pain-relieving cream/topical to affected area 2 to 3 times per day
- Multivitamin with vitamin D
- Curcumin: 1,500 milligrams per day
- Fish oil: 2,000 milligrams per day (Some data shows fish oil may cause prostate cancer but may help prevent breast cancer.)
- Vitamin D_3: 1,000 units daily

Roll It Out

One of the very best ways to recover from a hard run is to give your aching muscles a deep tissue massage with a foam roller. These 6-inch-round, high-density training aids will cost you a fraction of what you'd pay to see a massage therapist, and work almost as well. Performed properly, rolling provides firm, constant pressure to the muscles and the deep connective tissue surrounding your muscles, tendons, and joints. It breaks down and releases the soft-tissue adhesions, scar tissue, and other toxins that can form when the muscle becomes inflamed—much like peeling through an onion—while also increasing blood circulation to the muscle and tendon areas to speed healing. The enhanced blood flow helps to keep the muscles long and pliable, so you don't feel so sore or stiff during your next run.

The most popular form of self-massage with the foam roller involves rolling the iliotibial band (IT band), which becomes easily inflamed with overuse. As it becomes increasingly irritated, runners complain of pain, or friction, on the side of the knee, usually a few minutes or more into their runs. Here are several exercises you can do with the foam roller to loosen those knots, whether in your IT band or elsewhere, and keep your muscles and tendons strong and flexible.

Iliotibial (IT) Band

✤ Position the roller just below your left hip and support your body's weight with your left forearm. Cross your right leg over your left, bending the right knee, so that your body is perpendicular to the roller and parallel to the floor. Slowly roll the entire length of your IT band on the foam roller, gliding back and forth from the hip bone to the knee.

✤ Perform two sets of 10 reps (1 rep is the equivalent of rolling down to the knee and back to the hip) on each leg, using your body's weight to apply pressure to the roller. Pause on an area for several seconds if you need to work out any knots. When first using the roller, it may feel like there's a knife cutting through your thigh. This is because your IT band is full of nerve endings. The pain should subside with more frequent use, but it's not a bad idea to ice the area for several minutes after rolling, which will eliminate any chance of soreness created by the deep-penetrating nature of the roller.

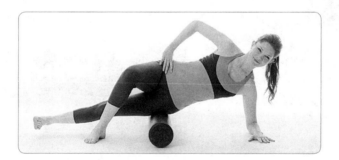

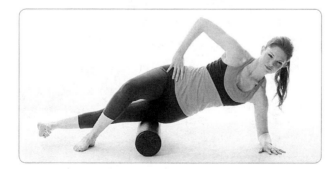

Hip Flexors / Quadriceps

✤ Lie facedown on the floor in a plank position so that your body is supported by your arms and elbows. Position your legs so the foam roller sits just above your knees. From here, roll your body down and up the roller slowly, from your hips to your knees, pausing for a few seconds should you come upon any knots. Roll for approximately 30 seconds, adjusting your legs to target other areas of the thigh if needed.

✤ If you want to work just one leg at a time, say your left leg, then cross your right leg over your left ankle and roll from the top of your thigh to your knee. Switch positions for the other leg. This will apply even more pressure to your quadriceps region and help to lengthen the hip flexors, the group of muscles responsible for lifting your knees while running.

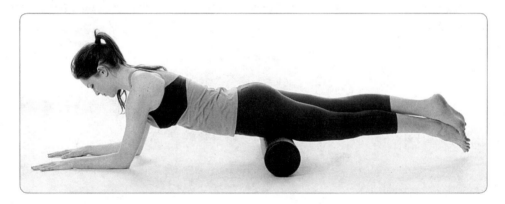

Glutes

✣ Sit down on the roller, placing your arms behind you and your hands flat on the floor for support. Position your body so that the roller sits under the back of your right thigh, just below your right glute. Cross your right ankle over your left thigh, and roll your body forward and back, making sure to hit all parts of your right glute.

✣ Roll for approximately 30 seconds and then repeat on your left side. The glutes are the big guns in running—they enable the hips to extend, which propels the body forward. They also do double duty as a decelerator, helping to stabilize your core and hips when your foot strikes the ground.

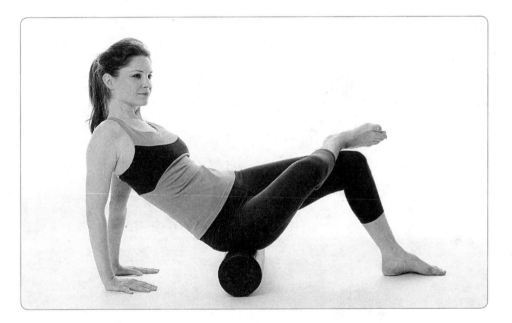

Hamstrings

✤ Start in a seated position with your hands flat on the floor, similar to the glutes-roll position, but with the roller positioned just above the knees. Lift your hips and roll your body forward until the roller is just below your glutes, and then roll back to your knees, or to the starting position. Roll back and forth for 30 seconds, adjusting your legs slightly to hit other areas of the hamstring.

✤ To increase pressure, cross one leg over the opposite ankle, which brings one thigh off the roller and targets one leg at a time. The hamstrings are responsible for the action of flexing and extending the knees, and they play a major role in transferring power between the hips and the knees.

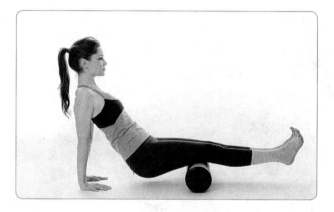

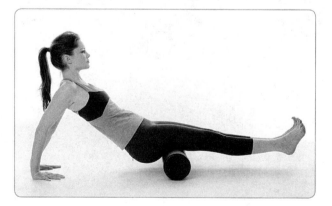

Calves

✤ From a seated position with your hands flat on the floor, move the roller so that it's resting just above your ankles. With the help of your upper body, roll your body forward until the roller settles just below your knees. Then roll back to the starting position. Roll back and forth on your calves for 30 seconds, crossing one leg over the other to increase pressure and work one calf at a time.

✤ The juncture of the calf and the Achilles tendon is an area that doesn't receive much blood flow, and rolling the calves is one of the best ways to boost circulation there and ward off injury. In addition to taking on the load of your entire body, the calf muscle's primary function is to lift your heel off the ground.

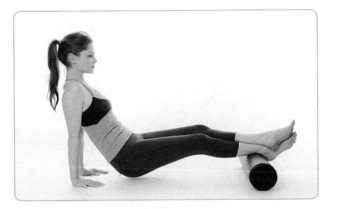

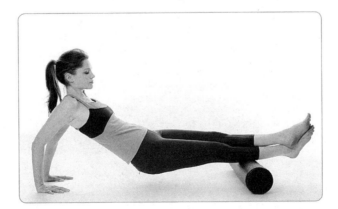

Injuries to the Lower Body (Below the Knee)

LORI, A 42-YEAR-OLD RUNNER, CAME TO SEE ME ABOUT 12 WEEKS INTO training for the New York City Marathon, complaining of pain in her right ankle. She said the pain had gradually worsened as her mileage intensified, and was almost unbearable when running uphill. I examined her and found that she had a severe case of muscle-tendon-junction Achilles tendinitis. She also had a condition known as pes planus (flat feet, or fallen arches), which no doubt contributed to her Achilles troubles.

I immediately shut her down in order to allow the tendon some time to heal—something that wouldn't have happened if she'd continued training for the marathon. A severe case of tendinitis such as this usually takes a minimum of 8 weeks to heal, and sometimes more.

During the first month of rehab, Lori traded in her running shoes for a form of low-impact cardiovascular exercise: a stationary bike. I also had her gently stretch the tendon as well as strengthen the muscle-tendon junction with some double-leg calf raises (page 61). To prevent a recurrence of any form of tendinitis, you must increase blood supply to the tendon (more on this shortly) as well as strengthen it, something I stressed with Lori. After the first 4 weeks, we substituted the elliptical machine for the bike and incorporated some single-leg calf raises (page 61) into her strengthening routine. At the same time, she took three 1-TDC esterified fatty acid tablets every morning, applied 1-TDC cream twice a day, and took fish oil and vitamin D supplements.

After 8 weeks, she was able to gradually ease back into running, without pain, which is a hallmark for any resumption of running. Lori still does the strengthening exercises to this day, and has gone on to run three marathons since without any issues.

She is one of the lucky ones, because while the Achilles tendon is the strongest, thickest tendon in the human body, it's very susceptible to injury. Every step you take transmits a force equal to your entire body weight through it—a force that is multiplied several times over when running. Considering the average runner takes approximately 160 to 200 steps per minute, the Achilles can take quite a bit of abuse over the course of any run, let alone a long training run.

It's no wonder why runners fear an injury to their Achilles, a likelihood that increases with age, since the tendon inherently has more watershed areas than most other tendons. Blood flow to these watershed areas is anything but robust, and as you age and the supply of blood to these areas diminishes even further, the tendon becomes more susceptible to tearing. Over time, the tendon becomes degenerative because it doesn't have the necessary blood and nutrients to repair the micro-trauma caused by running. It's like any other tissue in that it needs blood to restore and revitalize itself and maintain adequate health, but if you cut off blood flow to that tissue and don't get it the proper nutrients, the cells will eventually die.

In the case of many runners, the tendon can undergo some degenerative changes, causing the athlete to experience pain within the tendon. In medical circles, this condition is known as "tendinosis," although the layperson's term for it is "tendinitis." There may be some minor inflammation, but this is usually to the paratenon tissue, which surrounds the tendon. Tendinosis, or tendinitis, is an avascular condition brought on by a lack of blood flow to the tendon and its inability to nourish and repair itself.

Tendinitis is a very common issue with runners, and not just to the Achilles. You can suffer from posterior tibial tendinitis and tendinitis to the hamstring and hip, which we'll cover in the next two chapters. It can be prevented and treated if you take the right course of action. Here are some important prevention and treatment strategies for the Achilles and posterior tibial tendons, as well as some tips on how to combat some other common lower-limb injuries such as shin splints and plantar fasciitis.

Achilles Tendinitis

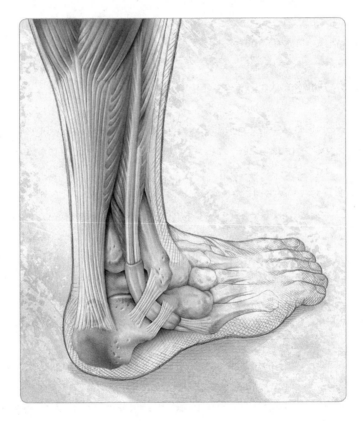

WHAT IS IT   Pain in the inner core of the tendon along the back of the ankle or heel. The Achilles tendon is the largest, strongest tendon in the body and connects both the gastrocnemius and soleus muscles to their insertion point at the heel.

It functions like every other tendon in the body to help absorb tension and also transmit power from the muscle (during contraction) to the bone so that the joint can move. During running, it serves to lift the heel off the ground, thus allowing you to push or toe off. Most micro-trauma to the tendon occurs at the muscle-tendon junction several inches above the heel or to the watershed areas within the tendon.

WHAT CAUSES IT   The Achilles has watershed areas within the tendon that receive very little blood supply, thus making it very difficult to repair any repeated micro-trauma that occurs to the inner core of the tendon.

The presence of blood in these watershed areas diminishes even further with age, thus increasing the risk of tendinitis, especially with overuse. A very small sub-set of the Achilles becomes inflamed, but it's the tissue between the tendon sheath and the tendon, also known as the paratenon.

SYMPTOMS   Runners with Achilles tendinitis will feel pain every time they lift their heel off the ground. In many cases, the tendon itself will feel very tender to the touch.

HOW TO PREVENT IT   Work on strengthening the Achilles and surrounding calf muscles, as well as your core. The very best strengthening exercises you can do for the Achilles are single- and double-leg calf raises. Start by doing gentle heel raises on a leg press machine, with little weight, and gradually transition to the more difficult standing one-legged variety. These exercises really keep the muscle-tendon junction strong and help fight off future incidents of tendinitis. Perform these calf raises after running, never before, and continue to ice the tendon at least two times per day.

In addition to anti-inflammatories and ice, consider adding heel lifts to your shoes when you return to running, as this will help to take some of the pressure off the Achilles. If several weeks of rest are needed, then get in the pool or do some cross-training on a bike or an elliptical machine to give your cardiovascular system a work-out and keep your endurance up.

HOW TO TREAT IT   If the pain lingers for several runs, then stop and take a few days off. Treat the pain with nonsteroidal anti-inflammatory medication, such as ibuprofen (if not contraindicated by your doctor), and RICE—rest, ice, compression, and elevation. Ice the area several times a day for 15 minutes. If the case is mild, and you caught it early enough, you should be back running again within a week or two at most. If it develops into full-blown tendinosis or chronic tendinitis, it will require about 8 weeks to fully heal because of the lack of blood supply. If you continue to run with tendinitis, then you increase the chances of a tendon rupture and surgery. In that instance, you can forget about running any races for a while.

The use of ultrasound therapy, which uses high-frequency sound waves to penetrate deep through your skin and direct nutrient-rich blood into the tissues to help relieve the inflammation, and electric stimulation therapy can also help speed up the healing process.

Posterior Tibial Tendinitis

WHAT IS IT   Pain and swelling on the inner side of the ankle. The posterior tibial tendon attaches to the back of the shinbone and runs behind and under the bony prominence at the lower end of the tibia. It provides support to the arch and the foot as you push off your toes, and assists in the flexion of the foot at the ankle.

WHAT CAUSES IT   Chronic degeneration in the tendon caused by a lack of blood supply; thus, when the tendon gets injured, it doesn't receive the necessary nutrients it needs to heal. Weakness or injury in this tendon can cause someone to gradually lose the arch and develop flat feet, or it can make a flatfoot condition even worse. When the arch collapses, it puts a tremendous amount of stress on the big toe. The spring action is gone, so the toe takes a beating and, in many instances, becomes arthritic.

SYMPTOMS   Pain is generally felt under the bony prominence on the inside of the ankle when pushing off. Much like plantar fasciitis, the condition can be very painful in the morning just after waking up or after sitting for a prolonged period of time.

HOW TO PREVENT IT   It's very important to keep the tendon strong, especially if you're flat-footed. Work with a physical therapist to develop an eccentric strengthening program for your feet, and make sure to incorporate calf raises into your regular workout routine. Runners with flat arches also tend to overpronate (excessively roll their feet and ankles inward) more than other runners and need a motion-control shoe to control the amount of pronation. Natural anti-inflammatories such as fish oil can also help.

HOW TO TREAT IT   Immediately stop running and substitute some low-impact aerobic activities like swimming and biking in its place for a few weeks. Ice the foot (with compression) at least twice a day for 10 to 15 minutes and apply a topical fatty acid cream, such as 1-TDC, to the injured area. When used as a topical, 1-TDC is highly transdermal and reaches deep into the muscle tissues and joints to provide instant pain relief. Nonsteroidal anti-inflammatories, like ibuprofen, can also help (if not contraindicated by your doctor).

Plantar Fasciitis

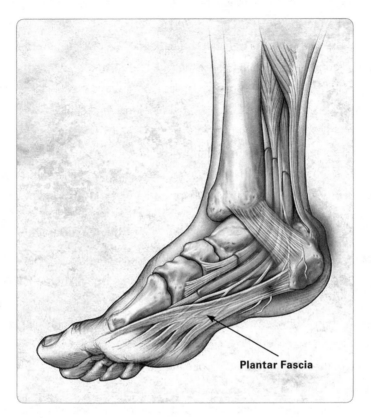

Plantar Fascia

WHAT IS IT A painful, inflammatory condition of the plantar fascia, a tendinous, flat band of connective tissue that stretches across the bottom of your foot and connects your heel bone to your toes.

WHAT CAUSES IT The plantar fascia's primary responsibility is to act as a shock absorber and maintain the arch of the foot. It helps to stabilize the foot upon landing and also assists in propelling you forward as you run. On contact with ground, the plantar fascia actually pulls away from its attachment at the heel bone—the medial tubercle. It tightens up and gets shorter, like a windlass mechanism in sailing, to absorb shock. When people have a biomechanical issue or something that affects how their feet strike the ground, such as a flat foot or a high arch, this mechanism is changed. There's a decrease in shock absorption to the foot and the ankle, which puts more tension on the plantar fascia as it's pulling away, causing micro-tears within the fascia.

Secondary plantar fasciitis can also be caused by a plantar fibroma (fatty cyst), which grows between the fascia and the skeletal structure of the foot to cause inflammation of the fascia, or a deep-surface partial-thickness tear to the fascia. Other contributing factors to plantar fasciitis include excessive running (overuse), particularly on hard or uneven surfaces, tight calf muscles, and wearing shoes with inadequate support. Walking or standing a significant amount of time in flat shoes, such as dress shoes, can also place more stress on the plantar fascia, says Dr. Rock Positano, director of the Non-surgical Foot and Ankle Service at the Hospital for Special Surgery in New York.

SYMPTOMS For someone with plantar fasciitis, the first few steps out of bed in the morning can be excruciating. Patients describe an intense, stabbing pain, as if they were stepping on a sharp rock, which usually goes away after 5 to 10 minutes, once the fascia has had a chance to stretch out. Runners with plantar fasciitis develop swelling inside the heel as they're sleeping, and when they put their foot down for the first time in the morning, they're pushing the fluid through a very inflamed area, which causes the discomfort.

Most people with plantar fasciitis develop it on the more dominant side (the right foot for right-handers, the left for left-handers), because there's generally more stress being placed on the lead foot, Positano says. It would be on the other foot only if you have a leg-length discrepancy or a knee, hip, or back problem that's forcing you to overcompensate.

Don't automatically assume that heel pain is plantar fasciitis, because it could be something else, such as a plantar fibroma or a heel spur (which is often caused by the plantar fascia pulling away from its attachment). Make sure you get the proper diagnosis so that you can treat your heel pain correctly.

HOW TO PREVENT IT Avoid wearing shoes that have little in the way of arch support. Dr. Positano tells his male patients to put a heel lift in their dress shoes, which takes a lot of stress off the plantar fascia and reduces tension where it inserts into the heel bone. If you have either a high arch or a flat foot, prescription orthotics will help to make your foot more biomechanically sound. Most important, if you're dealing with any type of foot issue, take a couple of days off and give the foot time to rest and rejuvenate itself.

HOW TO TREAT IT   As long as you're not dealing with a tear, stretching the fascia before you go to bed is a must. Sit up in bed with your leg straight and your knee locked, and drape a towel around the front part of the injured foot. Pull your foot toward you slowly until you start to feel a stretch in your calf. Hold this position for 20 to 30 seconds and do it three times on each foot before you call it a day.

Also cut back on your running and ice the heel twice a day for 10 to 15 minutes. Patients diagnosed with plantar fasciitis will typically be sent to physical therapy for treatments such as ultrasound therapy or electric stimulation therapy. Over-the-counter pain relievers, like ibuprofen, can also help (if not contraindicated by your doctor).

Metatarsalgia (Forefoot Pain)

WHAT IS IT   Pain and inflammation of the ball of the foot, typically felt near the rounded ends of the metatarsal bones (five bones in the forefoot located between the mid-foot and the toes). The condition is very common in high-impact sports like running, where the forefoot is exposed to repetitive traumatic forces.

WHAT CAUSES IT   Repetitive stresses on the forefoot from overuse (excessive running) can cause chronic irritation of the metatarsal bones and adjacent tissues, which absorb much of your body's weight during the toe-off phase of the running cycle. Much like plantar fasciitis, a runner's foot type can also play a big role. Those with high arches are more prone to developing metatarsalgia because they apply more stress to the forefoot when their foot strikes the ground. Flat, worn-out shoes with poor forefoot cushioning and support can also contribute to metatarsal problems.

SYMPTOMS Patients complain of symptoms very similar to those of plantar fasciitis, except in the forefoot—many have the sensation that they're walking on marbles. A number of different foot maladies can contribute to symptoms that are similar to metatarsalgia and can cause a great deal of forefoot pain. The first involves the deep transverse metatarsal ligament, a narrow band that connects the heads of all five metatarsal bones. The repetitive motion of running can really beat up this ligament, also known as the plantar plate, causing degeneration and tearing in the ligament. An ultrasound or MRI should be able to pinpoint any deformities or signs of inflammation in this ligament.

The aforementioned diagnostic tests should also be able to spot a neuroma, or growth of nerve tissue, which can become irritated and inflamed with repetitive running. Runners with a neuroma typically describe a pain that radiates into their toes, or a burning sensation or numbness in the front of their foot. It may feel as if they're walking barefoot on stones, and some patients speak of having to take off their shoes and rub their foot to make it feel better.

The final forefoot agitator is extremely common with runners and involves the two sesamoid bones under the big toe. What's tricky about these two little bones is that they're enmeshed in the middle of a tendon—they're encapsulated by the flexor hallucis brevis tendon, one of several tendons that exert pressure from the big toe against the ground and help initiate the act of walking. The sesamoids are solely responsible for propelling a person forward, and when these become inflamed because of repetitive trauma or even a stress fracture (a condition known as sesamoiditis), it can become a very painful problem for runners.

HOW TO PREVENT IT Some sports medicine hospitals and facilities, such as the Hospital for Special Surgery, have a high-resolution motion/gait analysis system known as a MatScan, which looks at how your forefoot distributes weight and exerts pressure as it contacts the ground. This can be a very helpful diagnostic tool in preventing metatarsalgia and forefoot pain, as can an X-ray, MRI, or ultrasound. Dr. Rock Positano says that runners with a history of forefoot pain should definitely get an X-ray taken of the ball of their foot to see if any of the metatarsal bones are plantar-flexed (in other words, naturally inclined to drop down a little more).

HOW TO TREAT IT   Positano, a podiatrist, is very high on prescription orthotics as a way of protecting the bones, ligaments, tendons, and other structures that make up the foot. "They're like prescription eyeglasses for the foot," he says. "What they basically do is address the mechanical deficiencies present in the foot and ankle, help to reinforce areas that are weak so that the foot doesn't have to work as hard, and reduce the stresses that go through the foot. They also make your feet better shock absorbers, which helps protect the knees, hips, and back."

Not every patient needs foot orthotics, however. Metatarsal pads and other shock-absorbing insoles can provide comfort and support to your forefoot. Icing the inflamed area for 10 to 15 minutes twice a day can also provide relief, as can making sure that your shoes have adequate padding in the forefoot and are appropriate for your foot type. Runners with a high arch typically supinate when they run and need a well-built-up cushioning shoe, which will encourage them to pronate more naturally.

Shin Splints

WHAT IS IT   The medical term is "medial tibial stress syndrome." Runners know it as dull ache in the lower part of the leg, just behind or on either side of the shinbone (tibia).

WHAT CAUSES IT   Excessive overloading on the bone and the muscle-bone interface, often brought on by a sudden increase in mileage. Beginning runners and those who return to running after taking several months off are prone to getting shin splints. Too much weight can also play a factor, as can poor biomechanics (excessive pronation), weak and inflexible calf muscles, running on hard or uneven concrete surfaces, and poorly cushioned shoes. Low bone density is also an issue, especially among postmenopausal females, who must be careful not to allow shin splints to turn into something more serious, like a stress fracture of the tibia.

SYMPTOMS Runners will typically experience soreness or tenderness when pressing on the muscular tissue lining the tibia. A tightening pain is generally felt after running for a short period and gradually gets worse. If you feel pain the minute you put weight on your lower leg, you could have a stress reaction or a stress fracture (tiny crack) in the bone itself. It can be difficult to differentiate shin splints from a stress fracture, but if you do a squat on the affected, weight-bearing leg and it aches, then you more than likely have a stress fracture.

HOW TO PREVENT IT Increase your mileage gradually, especially if you're just starting a training program or getting back into running. "Your body responds better if you slowly build up volume and intensity," says Dr. Joseph Feinberg of the Hospital for Special Surgery. "If you do something too suddenly, then the tissue doesn't have a chance to respond and regenerate, which causes injury."

Cushioning is very important too. When the outsoles on your shoes start to smooth over, like a bald tire, it's time to get a new pair. Make sure that your shoes support the proper foot biomechanics, especially if you need to get your overpronation under control. Stretching your calf muscles prior to running may also help protect the tibia and surrounding muscle tissue from getting overloaded. Last, consider wearing a compression sleeve or legging over your lower leg, which hugs your body and is believed to increase circulation in the affected area, as well as provide more support and better shock resistance.

HOW TO TREAT IT At the very first sign of shin pain, make sure to ice the area. Instead of just putting an ice pack on it, apply an ice cube or two directly to the shin and use it to gently massage the shin and surrounding tissue, Feinberg says. This combination of ice and soft-tissue massage helps reduce swelling and inflammation around the tibia and simultaneously increases blood flow to the area to speed up healing. Prescription orthotics and motion control shoes can help correct existing biomechanical issues, such as overpronation, as well as provide more arch support and cushioning.

Stress Fracture

WHAT IS IT   A crack in the bone often caused by a rapid increase in training and excessive loading on the bone. The most common stress fractures in runners occur to the foot (metatarsal bones, heel bone), tibia (shinbone), and hip.

WHAT CAUSES IT   Think of a stress fracture like the federal budget deficit: Bone is a live tissue that is constantly broken down and built back up, and when there is a deficit (i.e., more breakdown than buildup), a stress fracture occurs. Increasing the volume and intensity of your training can lead to this deficit, as can overworking the bone by applying force to it over and over again. Runners may also develop a stress reaction, or weakening of the bone, which can morph into a stress fracture.

SYMPTOMS   Most patients complain of pain in the foot, shin, or front of the groin that worsens with running or walking. Performing a single-leg stand will also cause significant pain in one of these three areas. The bone affected will be tender to the touch.

HOW TO PREVENT IT   Avoid increasing your mileage by more than 10 percent from week to week; build it up gradually. Make sure to get your recommended daily allowance of calcium (1,000 milligrams) and vitamin D (1,000 units), both of which are essential to keeping your bones strong and healthy. If you're deficient in vitamin D, then your body won't be able to absorb the calcium it needs to rebuild bone tissue, which can lead to stress fractures. Strength training is also vital in the prevention of stress fractures, as it helps strengthen the bones and tone up the muscles, which act as the body's primary shock absorbers.

HOW TO TREAT IT   Running should not be initiated for 2 to 3 months after diagnosis in order for the stress fracture to heal completely. Rehabilitation should include pool therapy (using the water instead of weights as resistance), swimming, and biking to maintain endurance. With stress fractures of the hip, proceed with caution because of the lack of blood supply to the area. Some hip stress fractures need to be treated surgically.

Calf Strain

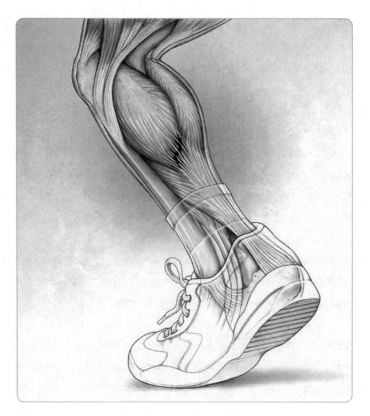

WHAT IS IT A tear to one or both of the calf muscles (gastrocnemius, soleus) on the back of leg between the knee and the heel. The primary job of the calf muscles is to lift your heel up off the ground so that you can push off the ball of your foot and propel yourself forward as you run.

WHAT CAUSES IT When the force across the muscle or muscle-tendon junction becomes too great, it can create a tear in the muscle fibers. The muscle gets over-stretched, which can happen when the foot pushes off the ground too violently or when you suddenly change directions or running surfaces (from the sidewalk to the street, for example). Another major contributor to muscle strains is dehydration. The body loses a lot of sweat during running—particularly in the summertime or in extremely hot conditions—and if the muscle cells don't get enough water and sodium (electrolytes), it can lead to abnormal contractions, cramping, and strains.

SYMPTOMS   Patients generally complain of pain and stiffness in the calf while stretching and running. Some may experience a sudden tearing sensation when first injuring the muscle. Depending on how severe the tear is, there may be swelling or bruising in the area and the muscle can be tender to the touch. It may be difficult to put pressure on the affected leg or walk without a limp.

HOW TO PREVENT IT   Stay well hydrated, particular in hot conditions when you're prone to sweating more. Make sure to consume an adequate amount of electrolytes, in particular, sodium. Water alone will not replace the salt you dissipate in your sweat. Strengthen the calf muscles eccentrically with heel raises (make sure your muscles are warm first), and avoid running on uneven and very hard surfaces. Wear shoes with adequate support and cushioning to take some of the load of the Achilles tendon and calf muscles.

HOW TO TREAT IT   If the damage is mild (known as a Grade 1 strain), then apply ice to the affected area several times per day for 15 to 20 minutes and avoid one-legged activities like running until you regain full strength or range of motion in the injured muscle. You should be able to resume running in 1 to 2 weeks, if not sooner, although if there's more extensive damage to the muscle fibers (a Grade 2 strain), it may take 3 to 4 weeks to heal. Apply 1-TDC fatty acid cream to the area to help reduce inflammation in the muscle tear and speed the healing process. Natural anti-inflammatories such as vitamin D (1,000 units per day) and fish oil (2,000 milligrams per day) can also help enhance recovery, as can deep-heat ultrasound therapy.

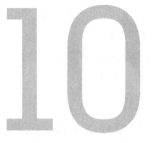

Injuries to the Knee and the Thigh Area

LIKE MOST FIRST-TIME MARATHONERS, RICH HAD A GOAL OF SIMPLY finishing the New York City Marathon. The idea that he would get hurt never entered his mind. He was completely preoccupied with the challenge of running 26.2 miles.

Just 8 weeks into his training, however, Rich began to feel a dull ache on the outside of his left knee about 1½ miles into a 5-mile run on the treadmill. As soon as he stopped and jumped off the treadmill, the pain went away, but it returned about a mile into his next run in Central Park. Like many competitive runners, Rich chose to ignore the pain in hopes that it would disappear, but it continued to get worse and worse, to the point where he couldn't run any more once it started.

Rich was diagnosed with inflammation of the iliotibial band, or iliotibial band syndrome (ITBS), a very common running injury often associated with increasing your mileage too much and too quickly during training. Rich never even knew he had an IT band (a thick tissue that runs along the outside of the thigh), but experienced runners know that ITBS can creep up from time to time like a very bad cold. For

Rich, it caused him to postpone his first marathon until the following year, when he ran without any IT pain whatsoever.

Here's a more in-depth look at ITBS along with some other common running injuries related to the knee and thigh.

Iliotibial Band Syndrome (ITBS)

WHAT IS IT The iliotibial band is a thick fibrous tissue that runs along the outside of your hip and thigh, and attaches to your shinbone (tibia) just below the knee. Its function is to stabilize your legs—mainly, the four quadriceps muscles at the front of each thigh whose job is to flex and extend your knees. Without the support of the IT band, your legs would move all over the place, and you'd have a hard time standing, let alone running.

WHAT CAUSES IT While not as strong as your Achilles tendon, a well-functioning IT band is like a bungee cord, very pliable and tough. However, it can be very susceptible to micro-trauma (mini-tears) within the tissue, due to overuse and a poor supply of blood flow to the area. Repeated micro-trauma to the IT band causes fibrotic changes in the tissue, which can cause the band to become more rigid, like a piece of gum that's been chewed too much. As the knee flexes and extends during running, the poorly functioning IT band becomes increasingly less flexible and more irritated, which is why most runners don't normally experience the first onset of IT pain until a mile or two into their run.

People at risk of getting ITBS are those who overpronate—as the excessive inward rolling of the feet puts additional stresses on the band—and those with flat feet, bowlegs, a leg-length discrepancy, or a pelvic malalignment. Weak hip abductors can also contribute to ITBS, since these muscles on the outer thigh work in conjunction with the IT band to help stabilize the knee joint. People with sciatica (a compression of the spinal nerves in the lower back and buttocks region) are also prone to ITBS, as this condition causes the hip abductors and tensor fasciae latae (TFL) muscles to weaken, further stressing the IT band. The TFL muscle, which connects to the IT band about two-thirds of the way up the thigh, is especially important to the proper functioning of the IT band, since it allows the band to stretch. The weaker it is, the less supple the IT is, and the more likely it is to become irritated.

SYMPTOMS   Patients generally complain of pain on the outside of the knee, where the IT bends over the knee joint and is stressed the most. Some people will also experience IT pain on the outside of the thigh, but it's usually less severe than the irritation felt on the side of the knee.

In few instances, the IT band may rub or snap against the outside part of the knee when it goes from flexion to extension, but more often than not, the pain is a result of micro-trauma to the tissue fibers. This pain will often get worse when running down hills or stairs, since running this way forces the IT to work harder to stabilize the knee. Conversely, the pain may subside the moment you stop running and start walking, since the latter puts less stress on the IT band; in running, one leg bears most of your weight every time a foot strikes the ground, whereas when walking, your weight is more evenly distributed over both, which helps alleviate pressure on the IT.

HOW TO PREVENT IT   The trouble with IT band syndrome is that most runners have to suffer through it once or twice before they even recognize what it is. Only then, once they've been diagnosed or done some research of it on their own, can they begin to know how to prevent it. If you're reading about ITBS for the first time, there are some basic steps you can take to prevent it.

First, make sure your shoes have enough arch support, especially if you tend to overpronate. Second, try to run on flat surfaces whenever possible. If you have to run on the side of the road, then make sure to alternate the direction you run every other day. Most roads are cambered, which means they're higher (and flatter) in the center and slope off on either side; thus, when you run on the edge of the road, your pelvis is tilted and one foot is lower than the other. Such biomechanical malalignments can predispose either leg to ITBS.

Strengthening the IT band and the neighboring hip abductor and TFL muscles (see the standing leg kicks and monster walk exercises in chapter 5) is also extremely helpful, as is stretching the IT band. Not everybody believes you can stretch it, but I'm not in that camp. Yes, it's thick and very sturdy, but it's not made of steel. You need to keep it as elastic as possible, and the best way to do that is to stretch and roll it.

A foam roller helps to break down soft-tissue adhesions and scar tissue, and it also increases blood circulation to the injured muscle or area to speed healing. The roller has become synonymous with both preventing and treating ITBS, as it offers the same benefits as a deep, penetrating sports massage but at a fraction of the cost. To learn how to roll your IT band, refer back to the foam roller exercises in chapter 8.

HOW TO TREAT IT   If you start to feel the aforementioned pain on the side of your knee and it persists for several days, then stop running. Head home and immediately apply ice (with compression) to the injured area for 15 minutes. If you own a foam roller, then massage the leg on the roller before applying the ice. This is important: Rolling the IT band will stimulate blood flow to the area, which encourages healing by flushing bad toxins away from the affected tissue, but it will also bring about inflammation, and you don't want that inflammation, or soreness, to linger. This is why you should roll first and ice second. The ice constricts the flow of blood to the area, causing the swelling to subside. Then, once the ice is removed and the area begins to warm up, new blood comes gushing in, once again carrying away the bad toxins.

Besides foam rolling and ice therapy, I recommend taking a fish oil supplement (2,000 milligrams per day) with vitamin D. Recent studies have shown that the omega-3 fatty acids—EPH and DPH—found in fish oil supplements are safer and equally as affective at combating inflammation as ibuprofen and other non-steroidal anti-inflammatory drugs (NSAIDs). Topical creams such as Aspercreme or those containing CMO (cetyl myristoleate), which is rich in fatty acids, also help speed recovery because of their ability to penetrate deep under your skin.

Continue to perform your IT strengthening and flexibility exercises while you're rehabbing. If you're in the middle of a marathon-training regimen, maintain your endurance by exercising on the elliptical machine, which is very low impact. Or try water jogging: Suspend yourself on a noodle so that your feet are not touching the bottom of the pool, and move your legs back and forth in a fast walking or slow jogging motion. Do this for 30 minutes to 1 hour and you'll really get a cardiovascular workout, without putting any stress on the IT band.

Do not return to running until you have full, pain-free range of motion in the affected area. How long that will take depends on the individual, but you should shut yourself down for at least a week upon the first onset of IT pain. After a week, ease yourself back into running: Start with 30 percent of your normal mileage, then increase it to 50 percent 2 to 3 days later, then 70 percent, and finally 100 percent. If at any point the pain resurfaces, then stop and get yourself to physical therapy. Your therapist will likely treat the injured area with ultrasound (using high-frequency sound waves to help to relieve the inflammation).

If physical therapy doesn't work after an extended period of time, then you should see a specialist. He or she might give you a platelet-rich plasma injection—known as PRP—in which blood is drawn from the patient, spun down (i.e., enriched with platelets), and then reinjected back into the damaged area, accelerating tissue repair and regeneration. I've had great success using this technique on a number of my ITBS patients. In most instances, they return to normal activity within 2 weeks, with no painful symptoms.

Runner's Knee (Patellofemoral Syndrome)

WHAT IS IT Pain in the front part of the knee associated with the patellofemoral joint, one of three compartments in the knee formed by the kneecap (patella) and front part of the femur.

WHAT CAUSES IT First and foremost, your knees take a tremendous pounding when running. The simple act of walking increases the load on your knee joints to one to two times your body weight, whereas running pushes it to four to six times your body weight. Running downhill multiplies it even more. Most of the time, however, front-of-the-knee pain is caused by a lack of overall core strength, particularly in the quadriceps and glute muscles. Flexibility can also be an issue in terms of tight hip flexors and hamstrings, and sometimes biomechanics are to blame. For every degree you overpronate, or roll inward on your foot, you externally rotate your tibia and internally rotate your femur. This rotational corkscrewing effect can lead to abnormal traction of the kneecap.

Women are more predisposed to front-of-the-knee pain than men because of the wider female pelvis and larger Q angle—the differential between the hip and the kneecap. The bigger angle causes the quadriceps muscles to pull on the kneecaps and thus causes abnormal tracking of the patella. Women also tend to have weaker hips and glute muscles than men do, and thus less stability in the pelvic region.

SYMPTOMS   Runners typically experience pain underneath or on the outside of the kneecap, most often when running downhill. When not running, patients will complain of front-of-the-knee pain when walking up and down stairs, bending at the knees, or sitting for prolonged periods (such as spending a significant amount of time in a car, plane, or movie theater where there's no room to stretch their legs). Many times the pain will cease with running but then return once the individual stops and begins to cool down.

HOW TO PREVENT IT   If you feel persistent pain in the front of your knee for a period of several weeks, go see a specialist. "If you can address this when it's a one-alarm fire versus a three-alarm fire, then you usually don't have to stop running," says primary care sports medicine specialist Dr. James Kinderknecht.

Once you're able to identify what's behind the knee pain, you should be able to address the source while continuing to train. Find time in your schedule for strength training, and pay special attention to your glutes—in particular the four hip abductor muscles on the outer thigh. These include the gluteus medius and minimus, which work together to pull your leg away from the center of your body and internally and externally rotate the thigh. They also help stabilize the pelvis so that you don't have too much internal rotation of the knee, which can increase loads on the kneecap.

Weak hip abductors can also contribute to a tight, poorly functioning iliotibial band, which can pull on the knee and cause patellofemoral pain.

Two of the best strengthening exercises for the hip abductors are the standing leg kicks (page 63) and monster walks (page 66). Avoid deep squats, lunges, or any exercise that puts an abnormal amount of stress on the kneecap. Modified single-leg squats (page 67) are okay, as are modified leg presses, where the range of motion is significantly limited.

Probably the most important step you can take in preventing runner's knee, however, is to simply not overdo it. Most training plans are several months long for a reason—to give your body time to adjust to the increase in mileage and intensity, and also to build strength and endurance. Taking on too much, too quickly, will only put you at a greater risk of injuring your knee. Follow the 10 percent rule: Do not increase your mileage by much more than 10 percent from one week to the next. Take it slow, and perform the three exercises above several times per week, either after you run or as part of your cross-training sessions.

HOW TO TREAT IT   Provided the pain doesn't make you alter your biomechanics in any way, you can continue to run. I recommend that you wear a Cho Pat knee strap, as it eases some of the load on the patellar tendon and the kneecap, which helps with both patellofemoral syndrome and patellar tendinitis. It's also vital that you keep the vastus medialis obliquus (VMO) muscle active and strong. This quad muscle can get shut down with patellofemoral pain, and it is vital to the functioning of the knee, as it controls the way the kneecap moves when we bend and straighten our knees. You can activate it through electric stimulation therapy or by pressing your knee down into your mattress as you're sitting in bed.

If the pain persists, reduce your mileage by 20 percent and apply ice to the kneecap (with compression) for 15 to 20 minutes several times per day. Take two or three Advil tablets with lunch and dinner to minimize inflammation in the knee (if not contraindicated and approved by your physician), and introduce more cross-training into your workouts. Be careful not to set the seat too low if you ride a stationary bike, as that can exacerbate your knee pain.

Knee Meniscus Tear

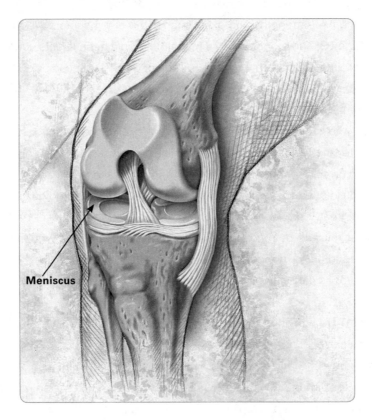

Meniscus

WHAT IS IT A tear of the meniscus, a very thin, rubbery piece of fibrocartilage that sits at the end of the bones in the knee and acts as a shock absorber between your shinbone (tibia) and thighbone (femur). Each knee has two menisci, which are triangular in cross-section and range from about 6 to 7 millimeters at the outside down to a thin point in the inside of the knee.

WHAT CAUSES IT Most tears of the meniscus in runners are degenerative, says Dr. Robert Marx, an orthopedic surgeon at the Hospital for Special Surgery in New York and a professor of orthopedic surgery at Weill Cornell Medical College. The meniscus wears down and gets very brittle, making it susceptible to tearing. In other sports that involve a lot of twisting and rotation of the knee joint, such as tennis, football, and soccer, a torn meniscus is more often the result of an acute injury, such as the knee turning too quickly with the person's full weight on it.

SYMPTOMS   While it depends on the severity of the tear, in most instances pain is felt on the inner or outer edge of the knee, not the front. If the pain persists during and after your runs, that's generally a good indication that something is wrong. Most meniscus tears are accompanied by swelling and stiffness, and you may have difficulty bending or straightening the affected leg. Patients sometimes have pain when they get up after sitting for a prolonged period.

Meniscal tears are frequently confused with patellofemoral pain (runner's knee), which is why if you're experiencing persistent knee pain, you should see a doctor to get a proper diagnosis.

HOW TO PREVENT IT   On rest/recovery days, avoid activities that require a lot of jumping and running, such as basketball, soccer, and tennis. Also stay clear of exercises that put a lot of stress on the knee, such as squats or lunges. Exercises such as standing leg kicks (page 63) and the standing tree pose (page 70) help strengthen and stabilize the knee, minimalizing the risk of a meniscus injury. Balance is very important, because the more unstable the knee, the greater your risk of a meniscus injury.

HOW TO TREAT IT   If the meniscus is torn, you can either remove it or repair it via sutures. Most degenerative tears are not suturable, because the tissue has deteriorated too much and you can't put it back together. Acute tears are much more suturable because the tissue quality is much better. If the meniscus is removed, it generally takes at least 4 to 6 weeks to return to running, and even longer (3 months) to return to training because of the volume of running. Standard physical therapy, including strengthening and stretching, is recommended. If your symptoms are not too bad, however, then you can opt out of surgery and treat it with anti-inflammatories (if not contraindicated by your doctor), ice, and rest.

After a scope and meniscal removal, there is increased risk of knee arthritis. So while it's okay to run one or two marathons after the surgery, competing in too many more will markedly increase your risk of developing knee arthritis—as will long-term running of more than 20 miles per week.

Knee and Hip Arthritis

WHAT IS IT   A loss of cartilage in the knee and hip joints. The most common form of arthritis is known as osteoarthritis, a degenerative condition caused by a gradual breakdown (wear and tear) of the cartilage that exposes more of the bone within the joint.

WHAT CAUSES IT   A 2013 study conducted by researchers at Queen's University in Kingston, Ontario, suggests that distance running is not as harmful to the knees as originally believed, and that it may, in fact, lead to less prevalence of knee arthritis later on. While that statement may be true—since runners tend to be thinner and have more muscle mass than less active people (muscles are primary shock absorbers which take pressure off the joints)—I have seen hundreds of times in my patients that that excessive running will tear up the knees, leading to knee arthritis.

Runners with a history of arthritis in the family are more predisposed to developing cartilage issues, as are those who play contact sports. A low, underactive thyroid can also put you at a greater risk of developing arthritis symptoms.

SYMPTOMS   Pain on the inside or outside of the knee when walking up and down stairs or running. Runners with hip arthritis generally complain of pain and stiffness in the hip with increased activity. They will often walk with a noticeable limp.

HOW TO PREVENT IT   While you can't prevent it, you can delay the onset of symptomatic arthritis by taking natural anti-inflammatory supplements like curcumin, fish oil, and vitamin D, and by maintaining an ideal body weight. Strength training also plays a vital role in slowing it down. Perform standing leg kicks (page 63) several times per week to strengthen the entire limb from your toes to your hip and to help establish better balance (proprioception) in the leg, which gets lost with arthritis.

HOW TO TREAT IT   Continue to take the above-mentioned supplements and pain relief medications such as ibuprofen (if not contraindicated by your doctor) as needed a few days a week. Avoid continued, excessive use of these NSAIDs, as they can cause kidney damage, stomach ulcers, and other health issues. Apply ice to the hip or knee for 15 minutes after you run, and 1-TDC fatty acid cream before and after you run; this safe-to-use anti-inflammatory cream penetrates deep to provide pain relief. For runners with knee arthritis, an unloader brace will help to take some of the load off of the affected compartment of the knee and provide more stability to the joint. As a result, you feel less pain and have more range of motion in the knee as you run.

High Hamstring Tendinitis

WHAT IS IT   Chronic pain felt at the tendon insertion, or origination point, of all three hamstring muscles. Also known as proximal hamstring tendinopathy, this type of hamstring injury is much more common in long-distance runners than strains or tears of the hamstring, which occur most frequently in sprinters or in those who play sports that require more explosive movements (pushing off the ground, changing directions), such as football, tennis, and soccer. A hamstring tear is an acute injury, whereas high hamstring tendinosis, (the medical term for tendinitis), is caused by a chronic degeneration of the tendon that all three muscles share.

WHAT CAUSES IT   The function of the hamstring muscles in running is threefold: (1) they decelerate the forward momentum of the striding leg as it approaches the ground; (2) they extend the hips to help stabilize the weight-bearing leg; and (3) they assist the calf muscles in extending the knee during the takeoff phase of the running cycle, helping propel you forward. They do a lot of work, and like so many other muscles and tendons in the body, are prone to wearing down with overuse. Repeated micro-trauma to the tendon combined with a lack of blood supply and healing causes pain within the tendon, particularly at the muscle-tendon junction.

Another contributing factor to high hamstring tendinitis may be the makeup of the muscles themselves, says Dr. Michael Fredericson, a professor of orthopedic surgery at Stanford University, and head team physician for the Cardinals. The hamstrings are composed largely of fast-twitch Type II muscle fibers, which fire much more rapidly than slow-twitch fibers, thus imparting more tension on the tendon with every muscle contraction. The hamstring muscles also spend a significant amount of time in a stretched position while you are running, which further increases the demands on the tendon.

SYMPTOMS Patients will complain of deep buttock or posterior thigh pain in the upper portion of the hamstring when accelerating at faster speeds, running on hills (especially downhill), or sitting down. The latter should come as no surprise, since the common point of origin for all three hamstring muscles is the ischial tuberosity, or sitting bones of the pelvis. The tendon that attaches to the ischial tuberosity becomes tender, making sitting very uncomfortable. Acute hamstring tears will typically be felt lower (mid-hamstring) in the belly of the muscle, and they occur when the force in the muscle is so great that the tissue begins to tear. These tears are accompanied by significant inflammation and swelling.

HOW TO PREVENT IT From a prevention standpoint, it's really important that you strengthen your core muscles, including your hamstrings, glute and hip stabilizer muscles, and abdominals, Fredericson says. A strong core will keep your pelvis in better alignment and prevent an anterior pelvic tilt from occurring, which is not good for the hamstring. In an anterior tilt position, the front of the pelvis drops and the back rises. Runners with high hamstring tendinosis often have this condition on the side they're experiencing the pain.

Since coaches started emphasizing more "eccentric" strength training exercises at Stanford, athletes on the football and track-and-field teams have had far fewer hamstring tears and injuries, according to Fredericson. "Eccentric" means that the muscle under tension is lengthening as it's contracting, and also braking at the same time (see page 59 for a more detailed description).

As with all running injuries, especially those specific to the muscles and tendons, it's important to avoid overdoing it. Increase the volume of your runs gradually, making sure to get plenty of rest and recovery between hard workouts.

HOW TO TREAT IT   The first thing you should do is undergo a physical examination to make sure your pelvis isn't in a malaligned position or that there aren't any other underlying conditions that may be causing the pain. If you are diagnosed with high hamstring tendinosis, start by getting soft-tissue massages to help break up adhesions and scar tissue and increase blood flow to the tendon, which expedites the healing process. You should also stretch the area regularly (but gently) until you regain normal range of motion in the hamstring. Strength is more important than flexibility in tendinopathy cases, however, so the key to your recovery is to progressively build strength in the tendon via an eccentric hamstring and core-strengthening program. Fredericson had an Olympic athlete who'd been struggling with this tendinopathy for several years, and following a program that consisted of hamstring stretching, soft-tissue mobilization, and eccentric strength training, was able to run competitively again within 6 months.

Some patients see great success with platelet-rich plasma therapy as well, which involves drawing blood from the patient, spinning it to enrich the platelets in the blood, and then injecting the blood back into the patient to stimulate healing or muscle regeneration in the injured area.

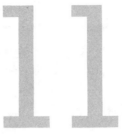

11

Injuries to the Hip and the Back

DOUG AND I HAVE QUITE A HISTORY TOGETHER. I FIRST MET HIM WHEN he was in his mid-40s, and he had just completed four marathons in a little over a year. A former sprinter in both college and high school, Doug came to me complaining of pain that radiated into his buttocks and hamstrings.

The root of his problem, however, was a mild hip impingement, which started to wear on the facet joints in his lower back, leading to facet arthritis. I injected Doug with cortisone in his facets and then followed that up with a radiofrequency denervation procedure that melted the nerve that carries the pain signal from the facets to the brain, thus eliminating the pain. "It was like an off switch, it was remarkable," Doug said.

It was also just the beginning of Doug's injury woes. A few years later, he was diagnosed with compressed, bulging discs between his L3, L4, and L5 vertebrae, mostly due to arthritis in his facet joints. "I'd get better and then it would just lead to another injury," said Doug.

When Doug turned 50, he started competing in triathlons as an alternative to running. His last marathon was in 2007 in Berlin, where he ran at less than full speed after tearing a calf muscle a month before, while tapering for the New York City Half. The facet problems also returned, but he'd get the radiofrequency treatment and be back biking and running before you knew it. This went on for several years, until he began experiencing hip and groin pain again in 2010, on his right side. It turned out he had a hip labral tear, to both hips no less, and he had surgery to correct both.

Doug, now 58, is the perfect example of Murphy's Law: "Anything that can go wrong will go wrong." He's also a good example of the evil that a degenerative hip condition can create, a phenomenon known as hip-spine syndrome. While the symptoms he presented to me early on suggested a back problem, the underlying cause was a hip impingement. This affected his biomechanics to the point that it started to irritate the facet joints in his back, leading to the arthritis. The hip condition was the trigger, and the butt and hamstring pain was the result of the secondary problem, the inflammation of the facet joints.

The good news is that with advances in medicine today and all the new treatments available, you can recover from these types of injuries and still run moderately for a long time. Doug is still competing in triathlons and continues to enjoy a very active lifestyle, thanks to many of the prevention and treatment strategies described in the following pages.

Here are the most common hip and back injuries associated with running:

Hip Impingement / Labral Tear

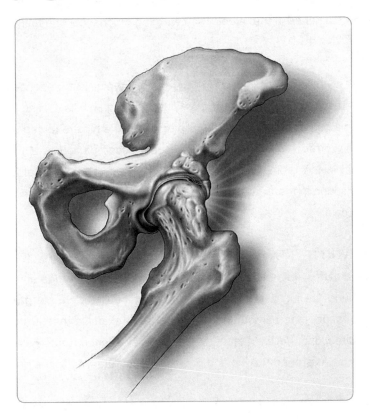

WHAT IS IT   Increased friction between the ball (femoral head) and socket (acetabulum) of the hip joint, which is known to cause pain in the groin. Also known as femoroacetabular impingement, or FAI, this gradual wearing-down action between the two bones can cause a tear of the labrum, which surrounds the outer rim of the hip socket. The labrum is a shock-absorbing fibrous cartilage, similar to the meniscus in the knee, which helps to protect the articular cartilage that lines the bones of the joint.

WHAT CAUSES IT   Imagine if you tried to drive an 11-foot-high truck underneath a bridge with a clearance of only 10 feet, 9 inches. You'd run into some trouble. This is essentially what happens to cause an impingement of the hip—there's a low clearance between the two bones of the hip, which causes them to bump into each other as the ball rotates in the hip socket, impinging the soft tissue in the labrum. The latter gets pinched in the middle, and with too much wear and tear, it eventually tears.

SYMPTOMS   With a hip impingement, runners will typically experience a dull ache in the groin area with prolonged sitting or when running on hills. Sitting in a very low seat (such as a car) or chair where the two bones of the hip are forced together can also cause discomfort. A hip labral tear is usually accompanied by a sharper, more localized pain in the groin. Frequently, patients will also complain of a clicking or catching sensation in the front of the hip. Performing a simple lunge movement will really cause pain.

HOW TO PREVENT IT   Make sure to stretch before and after you run (see chapter 7 for the best dynamic and static stretches) to help improve the range of motion in the muscles around the hip joint. The hip internal rotation stretch is a great FABERE (flexion, abduction, external rotation, and extension) exercise that stretches the hip in multiple directions. Perform standing leg kicks after each run to help strengthen the same muscles around the hip and provide greater stability to the pelvis.

HOW TO TREAT IT   Start with a conservative treatment plan involving rest, physical therapy, and natural anti-inflammatory supplements such as curcumin, fish oil, and vitamin D. Applying a fatty acid topical cream to the hip can also help to relieve symptoms. If none of these methods work, you may want to ask your doctor about platelet-rich plasma therapy. If the injury still doesn't respond, then you're probably looking at arthroscopic surgery.

Hip Tendinitis/Bursitis

WHAT IS IT   Pain on the outside of the hip associated with the hip abductor tendons—primarily the abductor medius—which help to move the leg outward, away from the midline of the body. A small tear in the tendon can eventually lead to bursitis of the hip—inflammation of the small fluid-filled bursae that line the outside of the hip and serve as a lubricant between the bones and the overlying soft tissue (muscle, tendons).

WHAT CAUSES IT Excessive running causes micro-trauma within the tendon that can't be repaired fast enough because of the lack of blood supply. A partial tear or weakening of the tendon is what leads to bursitis. The diseased tendon places more stress on the bursa as it glides over it (due to a change in biomechanics), thus triggering the inflammation.

SYMPTOMS Pain on the outside of the hip that increases with running or resisted hip abduction. The patient may also feel more pain when lying on the same side as the affected hip.

HOW TO PREVENT IT Avoid increasing your mileage too quickly or running on banked surfaces, which cause an unequal amount of weight to be distributed on one hip. Incorporate dynamic stretching before you run and static stretching afterward, and keep the hip abductor/glute muscles surrounding the hip joint very strong. Standing leg kicks (page 63) are great glute-builders, as are modified single-leg squats (page 67) and monster walks (page 66). Natural supplements such as fish oil, vitamin D, and 1-TDC (1-TetraDecanol Complex) capsules also help to curtail inflammation.

HOW TO TREAT IT Physical therapy should include exercises that both stretch the outside of the thigh and strengthen the abductor muscle-tendon junctions of the hip. The standing leg kick is the best exercise I know for strengthening the hip abductors. Ice the affected area for 15 minutes with compression at least two times per day, and apply an esterified fatty acid cream to promote better healing. I would recommend PRP therapy to help stimulate blood flow to the diseased tendon before getting a cortisone injection there. If you have bursitis, then you must also treat the underlying problem, which is generally tendinitis of the hip. Injecting cortisone in the tendon can cause tears and other problems, which may impede your recovery.

Facet Joint Arthritis

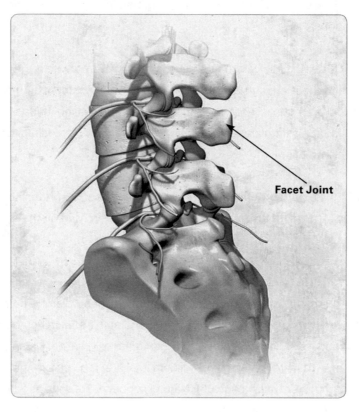

Facet Joint

WHAT IS IT A painful degeneration of the cartilage that cushions the facet joints in the lower back. These joints, located approximately two finger-widths away from your spinal column, are responsible for the flexion, extension, and rotation of the spine. Arthritis of the L4-L5 facet joint of the lower lumbar spine is most common among runners.

WHAT CAUSES IT The cartilage between the facet joints is very susceptible to wearing down. This process of wear and tear can be sped up if you are overweight, smoke, play a lot of contact sports, or run excessively. Any rapid increase in mileage or changes to your training regimen (such as speedwork) can aggravate the symptoms of facet joint arthritis and cause even more pain.

SYMPTOMS   Back or buttock pain that worsens with standing, walking, or running and difficulty standing up straight for a long period of time. The pain is often accompanied by a loss of motion and stiffness in the lower back and is typically relieved by sitting.

HOW TO PREVENT IT   First, avoid any rapid increases in mileage or changes to your normal training regimen. If you suddenly add 800-meter speed intervals to your training without conditioning your body for them first, you're going to beat up your facet joints, especially if you have a history of lower back pain. Take anti-inflammatory supplements such as fish oil, curcumin, and vitamin D as part of your daily routine, and keep your core and hip strong (see chapter 5 for exercises) to help relieve some lower back pressure. Try to limit your mileage to less than 20 miles per week; any more can have a negative impact on arthritis of the knee, hip, and facet joints.

HOW TO TREAT IT   Physical therapy should help restore some range of motion to the facets. Should the back not respond to these treatments, an epidural steroid injection into the joint is also an option, as is a procedure called radiofrequency denervation, in which the affected nerve or nerves are melted with a needle to stop them from sending pain signals to the brain. This procedure has been shown to eliminate facet joint pain for up to 2 years, based on clinical trial results.

Bulging Disc

WHAT IS IT   The spinal discs fill up the space between the vertebrae in your spinal column and act as shock absorbers to cushion the bones as the body moves. A bulging disc is a condition in which the soft inner material of the disc bulges out—like jelly oozing out of a donut—and presses on a nerve, causing pain in the lower back.

WHAT CAUSES IT   The load on the disc—often caused by excessive sitting or general wear and tear—becomes too much for the disc to handle, causing the inner nucleus pulposus to bulge out. Light jogging shouldn't aggravate this condition, although excessive running can put stress on the discs.

SYMPTOMS Patients may experience more back and leg pain with running, although pain is usually worse with prolonged sitting and during forward bending (e.g., sitting in a plane or car, bending over to tie your shoelaces). In some instances, a bulging disc can lead to sciatica and a feeling of numbness or pain that radiates through the buttocks and down the leg.

HOW TO PREVENT IT Get off your rear end and either walk, jog, or run at least 30 minutes daily. If you're working, then get up from your desk and walk to the water-cooler or go visit with a work colleague every hour. When sitting at your desk, prop your feet up on a stool, crate, or phone book to help relieve pressure on the discs. Take natural anti-inflammatories such as vitamin D, fish oil, and 1-TDC tablets to minimize inflammation on the disks. If you fly frequently for business, get up every hour and walk around the cabin.

HOW TO TREAT IT Cut back on your running and spend more time on the elliptical machine, a low-impact activity that will help you maintain your endurance while also keeping you on your feet. Avoid excessive sitting at all costs. If physical therapy, anti-inflammatory pain relievers (if not contraindicated by your doctor), and cross-training don't relieve symptoms, then you may need an epidural injection to speed recovery. Clinical trials also suggest that stem cell therapy can have positive results, especially as it relates to disc injuries and degeneration.

Miscellaneous Injuries

You're cruising along in the New York City Marathon when you make the turn into Central Park and suddenly your right thigh locks up. In excruciating pain, you manage to limp over to the sidelines and get medical attention for the cramp, but your dream of breaking 4 hours is shot.

This is a common fear among many runners—that they'll do a face plant in front of thousands of spectators because of a muscle cramp, or that they'll be hindered by a nagging case of side stitches that takes them several miles to work out. I would be remiss if I didn't talk about these two common conditions, because they can cramp your running style and cause major problems during a race. Here's what you need to know about both of these unpleasant and often untimely pains:

Muscle Cramps

WHAT IS IT A sudden involuntary contraction or spasm of a muscle that can last from several seconds to several minutes.

WHAT CAUSES IT Most muscle cramps are brought on by overuse and fatigue—you may be pushing harder or running longer than ever before, which explains why cramps are so prevalent in marathons. Dehydration also plays a factor, as does a low concentration of salt in the body. Some runners are very heavy, salty sweaters and don't take in enough of these vital electrolytes as they run, which causes the muscles to spasm.

SYMPTOMS When it happens, you know it. The pain can be excruciating at times, like nothing you've ever experienced before. The sensation is like that of being stabbed, except that the pain doesn't always go away immediately.

HOW TO PREVENT IT Run within your means. Don't extend yourself too much in terms of pushing your pace or distance, or running too much, too soon. If you're a salty sweater (you can tell this if you look at your face after a long run and you see a salty beard or raccoon eyes), then spike your sports drinks with salt tablets or make sure you consume a lot of salty beverages or snacks before you run. Many sports drinks are hypertonic, meaning that the concentration of salt is less than it would be in your own blood; in other words, they're diluted. Gatorade makes an electrolyte powder mix (Gatorlytes) that contains 780 milligrams of sodium, which, when added to your regular Gatorade sports drink, makes it more isotonic (i.e., equal in concentration to the sodium that's in your blood).

HOW TO TREAT IT Sometimes you can stretch the muscle or massage it to relieve the pain. In general, however, the best form of treatment is prevention: drinking a lot of salty fluids before, during, and after a race and making sure not to overextend yourself.

Side Stitches

WHAT IS IT   A sharp pain in your side, usually under the lower edge of the rib cage, which can make it difficult to run at normal speed.

WHAT CAUSES IT   There are a number of different theories, including that air is trapped underneath the diaphragm—the large dome-shaped muscle that separates the chest cavity from the abdominal cavity—but the most logical one seems to be inflammation of the diaphragm. When too much air gets trapped in the stomach, it pushes up on the diaphragm, causing what we know as a side stitch, or exercise-related transient abdominal pain (ETAP). These cramps often occur if you eat too close to your run, or after you take a long water break.

SYMPTOMS   Runners experience what feels like a sucker punch to their stomach, only it's on their side. The pain usually worsens with running, especially if they exert themselves more.

HOW TO PREVENT IT   First and foremost, don't eat too much before you run. Limit yourself to a small serving of carbohydrates, like a handful of trail mix or half a banana or energy bar (see chapter 4). On the course, drink smaller amounts of water or sports drink more often, as opposed to consuming 6 to 8 ounces all at once.

HOW TO TREAT IT   The best way to treat a side stitch is to stop running and take a short walk break, slowing down your breathing. Take several deep breaths and then resume running once the spasm disappears. People will often try to pinch their sides or change their breathing patterns, but the most effective method is to simply slow down.

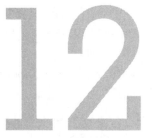

Training Dos and Don'ts

ANYONE WHO'S RUN A MARATHON WILL TELL YOU THAT THE ACTUAL race day itself is the easy part. I'm not saying that those last 6.2 miles won't be tough and that you won't be searching for every last ounce of energy your body has to give, but you have to do it only once. And your adrenaline is there to kick you in the butt when you need it. No, the hard part is simply getting there.

There's a saying among marathon runners that it's not about getting to the finish line; it's about getting to the starting line. It's about the lonely long runs in the heat of the summer when there aren't thousands of spectators there to cheer you on, and the 5-mile tempo runs in the middle of the week when you'd like nothing more than to be in bed or joining your friends for drinks. It's about fitting five or six runs into your busy schedule every week for months and not missing a beat in the other aspects of your life. It's about staying in on Saturday night before your long early-Sunday-morning run and resisting the urge to have that last piece of cheesecake just before you go to bed. Most of all, it's about getting out there and running when you simply don't have the urge or energy to do it. Not every run is going to feel great.

Training for a half- or full marathon is a grind both physically and mentally. As a runner, you must make a lot of sacrifices and be very diligent about not only how much you run and at what pace but also what you eat, how much you sleep, what you wear, and so on. It takes a tremendous amount of discipline and motivation. Sometimes 5 a.m. is the only time you can squeeze a run into your busy schedule—and I don't care who you are, it's not easy dragging yourself out of bed that early.

Physically, it might feel as if you're putting your body through an NFL training camp. The repetitive stresses on your muscles, tendons, and joints can take their toll, and if you train too fast or too much, you may find yourself watching from the sidelines come race day. And for any runner, that's a hard thing to swallow.

Every October, a parade of runners comes limping into my office because it's the peak month of training for the New York City Marathon. I like to call it the "October Surprise." It's when these runners are in full panic mode and trying to squeeze in more miles than their bodies can handle. Almost all the injuries I see are due to overtraining. My hope with this book is to put a stop to these aches and pains and to help you train smarter and more injury-free so that you can get to the starting line and then experience the thrill of finishing the race.

In this chapter, you'll find a ton of helpful information on how to get the most out of your training, as well as how to avoid the common mistakes that marathoners make in their training. Follow these rules, along with the marathon training schedules in chapter 13 or the half-marathon training schedules in chapter 14, and you'll not only stay healthy but also prepare yourself physically and mentally to run the best race of your life. While training for a half-marathon or marathon isn't all fun and games, it can influence your life positively in so many ways, from shedding a few unwanted pounds to improving your fitness, discipline, and concentration. Most of all, it will give you the confidence that you can run 13.1 or 26.2 miles and achieve whatever goals you might have, come race day. Here are several dos and don'ts for you to consider as you embark on your several-month journey:

▲ DO | Increase Your Mileage Gradually (The 10 Percent Rule)

A good rule of thumb, especially for beginning marathoners, is to not increase your mileage by more than 10 percent from the previous week. That means if you run 30 miles one week, you should run no more than 33 the next (30 x .10 = 3 + 30 = 33). In our Beginner's Marathon Training Program in chapter 13, the largest increase is 14 percent from week 3 to week 4 (29 to 33 miles), and that's in a 10-day week, or phase. The reason this 10 percent rule is so effective and widely adhered to is because it gives your body time to gradually adapt to the stress that comes from increasing the volume and intensity of your runs. You want to increase your mileage gradually from week to week, like an airplane taking off in flight. You don't want your mileage climbing rapidly, like a rocket shooting up into space.

"There's a constant breakdown and remodeling process that goes on, and as you build up more and more mileage, you want to give the body a chance to rebuild and respond," says Dr. Joseph Feinberg, the Hospital for Special Surgery's physiatrist in chief. "And you want to do that really slowly."

▼ DON'T | Try to Make Up for Lost Time

If you get injured or sick and have to miss a week or two of training, don't try to do that 20-mile long run your training plan calls for. Run a relaxed, easy 10 to 12 miles, or however many miles you can cover slowly in 1:30 or 1:45. Trust the training you've put in beforehand; don't go out and try to make up your mileage in a hurry just because your schedule says you should or you feel like you won't be ready otherwise. That's nonsense. A week or two lost due to illness or injury won't sabotage your marathon, but increasing your mileage too quickly will. The number-one cause of injuries during training is overtraining, and if you panic and try to rush back to make up for lost time, you'll be sorry.

▲ DO | Limit Your Long Runs to 2½ to 3 Hours

Running coach Tom Fleming says that there's no magic number when it comes to the long run, and that everyone's number is different. He prescribes to the theory that what's most important is your actual on-your-feet time, and not how many miles you run.

"If you were to just stand on your feet for 4 hours and do nothing else, you'd be exhausted," says Fleming, who ran 27 marathons each in under 2 hours, 20 minutes. "Now, can you imagine running for 4, 5 hours? That's what I tell beginning marathoners: You first have to learn how to stay on your feet for several hours. If I can increase your on-your-feet time and get you to run more, you'll have less of a problem trying to endure 42 kilometers when race day comes along."

There is a point of diminishing returns once you get past 2½ or 3 hours, Fleming says. His longest runs were 22 or 23 miles, although he did on occasion run 15 miles twice per day (30 overall). For an elite long-distance runner like Fleming, 22 miles doesn't amount to much more than 2 hours of on-your-feet time. But a beginning marathoner might need 2 hours to run 11 or 12 miles; therefore, running 18 to 20 miles would push them well past 3 hours, and that's too much time for any runner to be on their feet prior to the actual race day.

"That extra few miles on your feet could be the difference in fatiguing your bones, creating a stress fracture, or some other malady," Fleming says. "I happen to believe that 2½ to 3 hours is sufficient, especially in the course of a 10-day cycle when you're doing all that other running."

▼ DON'T | Set a Personal-Best Time on Your Long Run

Many runners feel the need to run at or very near marathon pace on their long runs, because it gives them the confidence they can do it again on race day. That kind of thinking is what leads to injury and personal anguish, not a personal best.

"I never saw the other side of 6 minutes during most of my training," says Fleming, who runs a 5-minute mile during his marathon races. "The average person preparing to run 42 kilometers, and maybe run a sub-4:30 or 4-hour marathon, needs to set a good distance pace first and then worry about the speed part."

Fleming recommends settling into a relaxed, easy conversational pace—one at which you can hold a conversation with a training partner—as you run about 60 to 90 seconds slower than marathon pace for your long runs. Better runners might shrink that down to 50 seconds. The speed, he says, will come from running and enduring all of those miles in training, and also from the number on your chest (i.e., adrenaline). "Train," he says. "Don't strain."

▲ DO | Train at a Variety of Different Speeds and Distances

The marathon training programs in chapters 13 and 14 will ask you to differentiate your paces, from relaxed and easy to steady to tempo to marathon race pace. Most of the runs will occur at a relaxed, easy pace, to build endurance, but if you want to optimize your performance come race day, then you need to incorporate some runs at race pace into your training. You also want to gradually get your body accustomed to running longer distances so that the first time you're asked to run 15 miles, you won't be in for a shock.

One of the best ways to go about both, Fleming says, is to run 2 to 3 miles at race pace in the middle of a medium-length run. For the more advanced athlete, running intervals (see chapter 6) at shorter distances is also a great option, as it teaches pace separation.

"You don't want to be running one kind of pace all the time," says Fleming. "Your body has to adapt to the amount of miles you're putting in, and it also has to adapt to what you hopefully can run 26.2 miles at."

▼ DON'T | Run Everything at Marathon Pace

While many beginners make the mistake of running all of their training runs at or very close to marathon pace, elite runners know that it's much more effective to train at a slower pace. "I found that the faster you are, the slower you train relative to your marathon pace," says Matthew Moran, Sacred Heart University's Undergraduate Exercise Science director. "And the slower you are in the marathon, the more you'll train at marathon pace."

Most elite athletes run 80 percent or more of their training runs at well below marathon pace, and only 20 percent or fewer of their runs at marathon pace. The average runner's split is probably more like 50-50, or even higher in favor of race-pace runs. They tend to run hard all the time, in part because they're so focused on their split times. Others simply don't know any better, or feel that running at race pace all the time will give them the confidence to do it again on race day.

The problem is that if you're running hard every time out, you're breaking down more tissue and muscle fibers than your body can repair, and you will break down. You also don't learn pace separation. You must be able to differentiate between relaxed and marathon pace so that you can properly pace yourself through the marathon. Chances are that if you run one speed all the time, you'll try to do it again in the marathon. You'll go out too fast and try to hang on, versus gradually getting faster, which is called a "negative split"—running the second half of a race faster than you did the first half. It's a strategy used by many experienced long-distance runners who feel it's best to conserve their energy during the first half of the race so that they feel rested and stronger for the stretch run, rather than tired and fatigued.

"I want everyone to run progressively, starting at, say, 9:30 [pace], then 9:20, then 9:10," Moran says. "You might run a few miles at marathon pace during a 6- or 7-mile run, but you're probably going to average a little slower than marathon pace. This is really the way you should run a marathon, at negative splits. Every chance you have to go out and run should be a chance for you to practice running a marathon in the correct way."

▲ DO | Rest and Go Easy After a Long Run

If the long run is the number-one most important part of your training, and I believe it is, then number one-A is the recovery. The average runner needs approximately 2 days, or 48 hours, to recover from a long run of 18 miles or more. That gives your body sufficient time to repair and rebuild itself. If you run hard the very next day following your long run, you build up more tiny micro-tears to the muscles than you can fix. You also don't give your bone tissue enough time to turn over and remodel itself, which can lead to stress fractures.

I'd rather you rest too much than not at all. While you might be able to run every day in your 20s, you'll feel better and run stronger if you give yourself one or more easy recovery days after every long run. This is especially true for baby boomers and runners over the age of 40, because as you get older, there is less blood supply to the muscle-tendon junction and a greater risk of injury with over-training. In our marathon training plans in chapter 13, all long runs are followed by a day off and an easy recovery run at a pace 50 to 90 seconds slower than marathon pace. This easy effort helps increase blood flow to the damaged muscle fibers, delivering fresh oxygen and nutrients to the muscles so that they can repair themselves and come back even stronger.

Always remember to stretch immediately after your long run, as this will also increase blood flow and speed up recovery. As you're stretching, replenish your muscles with a post-workout recovery drink high in electrolytes, carbohydrates, and protein. Low-fat chocolate milk is an excellent option, as it has the same amount of electrolytes as many sports drinks and double the amount of carbo-hydrates and protein. It also contains calcium to help restore your bones back to health. In hot, humid weather, electrolyte-rich all-natural coconut water is a great rehydrating recovery drink.

▼ DON'T | Train Hard the Day Before a Long Run

Just as you should go easy the day after a long run, you should be taking it fairly slow the day before—especially the day before a marathon or half-marathon. "I never went to a mall for 20 years," Fleming says, "because I didn't want to kill my legs. You get these marathoners from out of town who come to New York and walk around the city all day long on Saturday. . . . And they wonder why their legs are dead on race day?"

Some coaches recommend running the day before a long run at tempo or race pace, because it does a better job of simulating the fatigue you'll feel in a marathon. For the advanced runner, I think this is okay, but for the beginning marathoner, you need to preserve your energy as best you can for the big run ahead of you. Take in a movie or a show, or spend the day relaxing and enjoying a book. For you intermediate runners, go ahead and run 4 or 5 miles, but do so at the same easy, relaxed pace as your long run. Avoid any hilly terrain that could fatigue your legs too much.

▲ DO | Use Your Long Run as a Dress Rehearsal

The long run is not only an endurance-builder; it's your best opportunity to practice, or simulate, what goes on in the marathon. This is the perfect time to try different energy gels, chews, and sports drinks to see what your body can stomach and what it can't. It's also a good time to practice a hydration strategy for the race, meaning how often you'll stop to consume water and electrolytes. Fleming recommends that you try to run at least one mid-long or long run in both hot and cold weather. You never know when extreme weather is going to pop up, as it did at the 2012 Boston Marathon, when temperatures soared into the upper 80s. If you have a plan in place for such conditions (for example, consuming more electrolyte-replacement drinks and tablets on extremely hot days) and have had a chance to simulate it beforehand, you'll be much better prepared.

Your long run also provides you with an opportunity to practice your race-day strategy, at least in the very beginning. Many runners start out too fast and then try to hang on in the marathon, which is usually a very unsuccessful strategy. Since your long runs are conducted at a very slow, conversational pace, you should know how to run relaxed and easy at the start of your race. You also want to make sure you're consuming a sufficient amount of carbs (but not to the exclusion of other foods) the week of your long run, and you should test to see which foods are most easily digestible, both the night before and the morning of your long run.

▼ DON'T | Wait till the Marathon to Try GU for the First Time

You don't want to be in for any unpleasant surprises come race day, so if you've never tried GU or energy gels before, don't start now. Stick with what you know works, and stay away from anything you haven't tried before. You don't want to withdraw from the race with a sudden tummy ache that you could've avoided. The same goes with what you put on your body. If you want to try out a new pair of socks or a compression shirt that a friend recommended to you, then take them for a test drive during one of your long runs, but not on marathon day.

▲ DO | Keep a Journal or Training Log

You learn more about yourself with every run, which is why it's helpful to keep a daily training log or diary. (You can also join an online social running site, such as Dailymile, RunKeeper, or MapMyRun, which allows you to track your workouts, make comments, and interact with friends.) Each entry should include the loop you ran, the distance, your time, and most important, your own evaluation of the run. Did the pace feel relaxed and easy to you, or was it too hard? Did the distance feel like too much, or could you have run another 3 or 4 miles? Jot down anything that was out of the ordinary or that caused you to feel anxiety or distress—for example, if you felt some stiffness in your Achilles tendon when you ran on a particularly hilly or sloped part of your route. If you found a particular song or two or a playlist that energized you for your run, make a note of it.

After a while, you should be able to easily identify what you're doing right and wrong in your training. You'll learn what workouts you like the best and the least, and what you should and shouldn't eat before your training runs. You'll also be able to see the steady progression you're making in the volume and effort/intensity of your runs, which should boost your confidence as you near your big day.

▼ DON'T | Let the Journal Keep You

Some people are obsessed with putting miles in their book, but little of anything else. They think that the miles are all that matters. Every part of your training should have a purpose, Fleming notes. If you're going to run an easy 7 or 8 miles, then it should feel easy and relaxed, and if it doesn't, then you need to ask yourself why. Perhaps you noted in your diary that your normal training pace earlier that week was a little too fast. Don't be a slave to your diary, but review your entries frequently because there's a lot to be learned from it, especially when you start preparing for your next marathon. (Yes, for you first-time marathoners, there's almost always a second marathon.) If you look back on your journal and think, "You know, I should've done more long runs," that's good. Now you can correct that mistake. But if all you ever do is track your mileage, you'll never be able to identify any mistakes to correct.

▲ DO | Find a Training Buddy or Join a Running Club

For more than 15 years, Joel Pasternack was Fleming's frequent training partner. He would be standing in front of Fleming's house in Bloomfield, New Jersey, come rain or shine, extreme heat or freezing cold. On the weekends, the two would be joined by several more runners for their training sessions in Brookdale Park. Fleming estimates that he and Pasternack ran more than 30,000 miles together.

"Their job was to get me tired, and my job was to take them apart," Fleming says of Pasternack and his other training partners.

When Fleming was having a bad day, Pasternack would stay 3 feet in front of him the entire time, encouraging him every step of the way. Fleming would return the favor by cursing Pasternack up and down. Pasternack took Fleming's hits without ever complaining and was a major reason for Fleming's success.

"[Having] the company made it a lot easier," says Fleming, who also trained frequently with Bill Rodgers, winner of four Boston and New York marathons between 1975 and '80. "It seems I always had a fresh set of legs to run with in the morning and afternoon."

Having a frequent training partner, especially for your mid-long and long runs, can really make a difference in your training. The miles tend to go by much faster when you're running with someone else, and it's also easier to run at a relaxed, conversational pace. Your partner should know all about your race goals and preferred pacing, and should rein you in if you start training too hard. You'll also be much more motivated to get up at 6 a.m. on the weekend if you know you have a partner, and not just your GPS watch or iPod, to keep you company on your 10-mile run.

▼ DON'T | Run with a Group That's Too Fast for You

If you join a running club or you're part of a weekly training group, stick to your pace group. Don't join the faster runners up front just because one of your pals is up there, or because your ego can't handle being in the last group. If you train too fast and too hard, you risk getting hurt, and then you'll really be embarrassed. Give yourself a couple of weeks to get acclimated to your current pace, and once that becomes very easy and relaxed for you, then progress to the next-fastest group. You should increase the volume and intensity of your runs very gradually, although you should be progressive in your training, too. By that, I mean if you're feeling really good, it's okay to run at a 15-second faster clip, just so long as you're relaxed and not racing.

Having a frequent training partner, especially for your mid-long and long runs, can really make a difference in your training. The miles tend to go by much faster when you're running with someone else, and it's also easier to run at a relaxed, conversational pace.

▲ DO | Start to Taper About 3 Weeks Out from the Marathon

Your last long run should occur approximately 3 weeks prior to the big race—not a week or a month before. This will give your muscles an adequate amount of time to recover from the hard training you've done over the previous 3-plus months. From this point on, you should reduce your weekly volume by about 25 percent each week, or phase, and also increase the number of easy runs in your schedule. In our Beginner's Marathon Training Program in chapter 13, the longest run in Phase 11 is 12 miles and all but one of the runs is easy. The mileage drops from 50 to 37 miles, and that's in a 10-day cycle. Our Intermediate Marathon Training Program calls for an even bigger drop in mileage, from 62 to 42 miles, and the longest effort is a mid-long run of 10 miles. In the days leading up to the marathon, the longest training runs are 4 miles, and the majority of them are performed at a relaxed and easy pace.

The taper is your reward for all the effort you've put in during training. It's an opportunity to get your body 100 percent healthy and ready to run on race day. Recovery is first and foremost during this time, and should be welcomed, not minimized.

▼ DON'T | Panic and Try to Squeeze in a Last Long Run

Just the mere mention of the word *taper* should leave you very excited. If it doesn't, and you fear that you need to get in another long run prior to the marathon, then you ought to consider deferring to next year or readjusting your expectations for the race. Two weeks—or less—is simply not enough time to get your body fully rested and prepared to run a marathon. You need to resist the urge to fit in another long run, because if you do, you risk getting hurt or fatiguing your legs to the point where they simply can't sustain a marathon race pace for 26.2 miles.

A lot of advanced runners become hypersensitive to their training during the taper, says Fleming. They want to do more because they're used to pushing themselves more. As a result, they feel the urge to run every day, which is fine,

Fleming notes, just as long as the volume is way down. You want to eliminate the more high-intensity workouts the closer you get to race day. Runners are worried about losing their endurance during the taper, and they shouldn't be— you're still actively running, but you're just not doing as much, so your body can rest and feel rejuvenated come race day.

The taper is your reward for all the effort you've put in during training. It's an opportunity to get your body 100 percent healthy and ready to run on race day.

▲ DO | Listen to Your Body

Runners are among the worst athletes when it comes to listening to their bodies. Short of a broken bone or a rupture of their Achilles tendon, they won't let anything deter them from getting in their training runs. Oftentimes they don't know they're injured until the doctor is standing in front of them with their X-ray or MRI results. If you feel a persistent pain in your Achilles, hamstring, knee, etc., for several days, and it's affecting the way you run and train, then stop and have a specialist check it out. It could just be that you need a few days of rest; it doesn't necessarily mean something is torn or broken.

▼ DON'T | Run Through Pain or Exhaustion

"Exhaustion" is a bad word. You should be training, not straining. If you're having trouble sleeping, you're constantly battling a cold, or your mood is often depressed, you may want to take a few days off from training. These are classic symptoms of overtraining, which is the number-one cause of injuries in runners. You should also be very wary of doing too much speedwork, especially if you're new to interval training. Mixing a high volume of running with fast speed can be a very dangerous combination if you're not adequately trained.

In college, Fleming once did a 15-mile training run in the morning when he had a dual meet in the afternoon. It was the only race he wound up losing in his college career. Common sense prevailed after that, and he scaled his runs down to 6 to 8 miles in the morning.

"I didn't sleep for 4 or 5 days I was so ticked off," he says. "But I learned my lesson: Your body needs to recover."

▲ DO | Leave Your GPS Watch at Home from Time to Time

Most runners are consumed by how many miles they're running in training, and at what speed. As a result, they lose sight of how they feel on their runs, since all of their attention is focused on their GPS watch and the times it's churning out. Do yourself a favor every now and then and leave the watch at home—and the iPod as well. Go for a 5- or 6-mile run on a familiar route, only this time look at the flowers and not at your watch, and listen to the birds and the *tit-tat-tit-tat* sound of your feet instead of the hard electric guitar chords emanating from your headphones. You'll become much more aware of your pacing, your breathing, and how your body feels. You'll also find it much easier to settle into a steady, relaxed pace, which is hard to do when you're constantly trying to achieve a certain split time on your watch.

▼ DON'T | Be a Slave to Time

Remember: The purpose of the training run for the average runner is to build endurance and on-your-feet time. The more consistently and gradually you increase your volume and the time on your feet, the easier the act of running becomes and the faster you become as well. Your body adapts to the stress of running more and gets stronger.

Most runners don't need speedwork to run a marathon, according to Fleming, even though they think they do. That type of high-intensity training should be reserved for the more experienced, advanced runner who is looking to shave 10 or 15 minutes off his or her race time. Yet, even for these runners, most of their training runs will be completed at an effort well below race pace. You should hardly ever run at marathon race pace on your training runs, and if you do, it should be for 2 or 3 miles max in the middle of a run (a mid-run pickup). Learn to run at a relaxed, easy pace and increase speed in your distance runs, says Fleming, and you'll find that your race goals are well within reach.

▲ DO | Run on a Moderately Flat, Soft Surface

Not all running surfaces are created equal; in fact, some are much tougher on the body than others, especially on your joints. The worst is concrete, which has very little give and is said to be 10 times as hard as asphalt. Some studies suggest that running on concrete for too long can break down red blood cells, decreasing your body's ability to carry oxygen and repair itself. Sand is another surprisingly bad surface to run on, because it's just the opposite of concrete—it's too soft. This puts you at a greater risk for an Achilles tendon, foot, or ankle injury. Many runners will choose to run on the firmer sand closer to the water, which is much better, but it also tends to be very uneven, or sloped.

So where do you run? Some of you may be limited in your options, especially those who live in urban areas and have to run on the sidewalks or edges of the road to avoid traffic. But whenever possible, you want to stay clear of concrete sidewalks and run on a more joint-friendly surface, such as packed dirt or gravel. Most big cities have parks or trails nearby that offer more medium to soft surfaces to run on. If you have dirt or grass paths or trails available to you, use them! They're much easier on your joints in the long run. Failing that, asphalt is much better than concrete—and faster, too.

The harder the ground below your feet, the more susceptible you are to overuse injuries in your training. Therefore, when you're scouting out possible running loops, look for a place that offers you a variety of different surface options. You don't want to avoid the asphalt entirely, since you're likely to be running on that surface in the marathon, but you'll reduce your injury risk if you limit your time spent on such hard surfaces.

▼ DON'T | Run in the Same Direction Every Time

Let's use Central Park as an example again: the preferred way to run in the park is counterclockwise. And since the running path is closest to the edge of the road (to allow water to drain off), it's also the most heavily cambered, or slanted. This slope puts a lot of uneven stresses on your body, in particular your downhill leg, which is bent slightly inward. That's why you want to always alternate the direction you're running in or the side of the street you're running on, so that downhill leg doesn't keep taking a beating. If the road or path you're running on is closed to vehicular traffic, then by all means run close to the center of the road, which is the flattest surface. But if that option is not available to you, mix things up to avoid running in the same direction every time. Not only is it safer for you, but you'll probably find it more interesting as well.

> Whenever possible, stay clear of concrete sidewalks and run on a more joint-friendly surface, such as packed dirt or gravel.

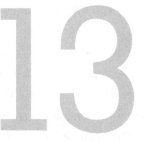

How to Run Your Best Marathon

WHEN I ASKED TOM FLEMING IF HE WOULD DESIGN THE MARATHON training schedules for *The New Rules of Running*, I explained to him that I was looking for a program that not only drew upon his experiences as a coach and former world-class marathoner but also incorporated much of the new science behind running. Above all else, I wanted it to be manageable and safe for runners, because in my mind, the best training program is the one that gets you to the starting line healthy. Chances are that if you get to this point, you'll be prepared to run your best race.

So when Tom brought up the idea of a "10-day-a-week" program, it made all the sense in the world to me. I mean, who says a training week has to be 7 days? With the extra 3 days, you can get more types of training in besides the long run, from an additional medium-length run to few different pace runs (i.e., relaxed, steady, tempo, marathon pace). Best of all, you can build in an extra day of rest or an easy recovery day. Most training programs don't provide for enough recovery time, in my opinion. And while the human body is an incredible machine capable of adapting to a tremendous amount of stress, if you subject it to too much, too often, it will backfire on you.

As you get older, into your 40s and beyond, you also need more time to recover from your hard runs. Your body simply doesn't respond to stress as it did when you were 25. Not only are your hormone levels diminishing, but there's also less blood circulating in the critical muscle-tendon junctions and lower limbs that absorb your body's forces when running. Therefore, if you're not getting an adequate amount of rest, you're not giving your body sufficient enough time to repair and rebuild itself, leaving you more susceptible to overuse injuries.

If you look at what's consistent in most 7-day plans, it's that you have an easy day prior to your long run and a recovery day afterward. You might have a day reserved for cross-training or speed intervals in there, but the traditional thinking is to follow a hard workout with an easy day or complete rest. So if you take the things that you know are consistent and build on them, does it really make a difference whether your program is 7 or 10 days? The answer is no. Our 10-day program adds up to 120 days, or just a shade longer than 17 weeks. Most traditional marathon training programs are either 16 or 18 weeks, and ours fits right in the middle.

There are simply too many advantages to a 10-day phase, or cycle, to ignore. Here are just a few:

More On-Your-Feet Time

In a 10-day phase, you can fit in a medium-length run in addition to your long run, increasing your volume of running without overstressing your body, thanks to the extra rest day. (Note: It may be an "easy" recovery day for the advanced runner.) These mid-long runs vary from as little as 6 miles in the Intermediate Training Program to a maximum of 12 miles in the Advanced Training Program. Generally, they fall between 7 and 9 miles.

The average runner underestimates the value of running more. This is evident in the times of today's marathons, because while runners may be faster at the very top, they're much slower overall. According to Running USA's 2013 Annual Marathon Report, the median time for male finishers in 2012 was 4:17:43, compared with

3:32:17 in 1980. For females, it was 4:42:58, nearly 40 minutes slower than 1980's median of 4:03:39. Granted, there were a lot fewer people running marathons back in 1980, especially recreational runners, but the numbers are telling. Even at the elite levels, the pool of sub-2:30 marathoners isn't as deep as it used to be.

"We had faster runners back in the 1970s because we did more running," says Fleming, who counts New York (twice), Cleveland, Los Angeles, and Toronto among his major marathon wins. "People ran farther. Sometime in the 1980s, it shifted to more quality miles—more speedwork—over quantity, and people started running slower."

In most intermediate marathon training plans, you won't be logging 39 miles in a week until about halfway through your training. But in our plan, you'll be approaching 40 miles in Phase 1. That's the luxury of having the mid-long run and the 3 extra days in each phase—it affords you the opportunity to run more, and in a way that won't tax your body any more than a 7-day plan would.

"In college I started running 110, 120 miles per week and went from being recruited by no schools to being an all-American," Fleming says. "I became good because I ran more—I slowly increased my volume without putting any attention on speed, and I became faster. If I can get you to run more, I believe I can get you to run farther and faster."

More Rest Time

Bill Bowerman, cofounder of Nike, and legendary University of Oregon track and field coach, trained more than 30 Olympians and 50 all-Americans by holding true to the hard-easy-easy philosophy of training that he developed in the 1960s—that is, you follow a hard run with one or more easy days to allow your body enough time to recover. By alternating hard and easy days, Bowerman theorized, you are able keep your body fresh so that it can exert itself again on your hard days. Your body's musculoskeletal and cardiovascular systems are able to adapt faster to the increasing stress of training, which makes you a stronger, faster runner. If you don't allow for sufficient recovery, however, then your body can't adapt quickly enough to these stresses and it breaks down, leading to injury or illness.

In Kenny Moore's 2006 biography of the renowned coach, *Bowerman and the Men of Oregon*, Bowerman is quoted as saying, "Take a primitive organism, say a freshman. Make it lift, or jump or run. Let it rest. What happens? A little miracle. It gets a little better. It gets a little stronger or faster or more enduring. That's all training is. Stress. Recover. Improve. . . . [But] you work too hard and rest too little and [you'll] get hurt."

In our 12-phase, 120-day training programs, each long run is followed by an off day—that goes for the Advanced Training Program as well. Every mid-long run is also succeeded by either an easy run (Advanced) or an off day (Intermediate), while our fast tempo runs—also known as race-pace pickups—are followed by an easy day. The idea is to provide enough recovery days so that your body can repeatedly tear itself down and build itself back up again. "Stress. Recover. Improve," as Bowerman would say. The 10-day phase allows us to do that, whereas in a 7-day week it's hard to get in the volume and intensity you need in training and still find the time to adequately rest and recover.

More Ways to Train

Your typical 7-day training week doesn't allow for many forms of training, outside of the weekend long run and perhaps some speed or tempo work early in the week. It generally consists of three or four shorter, mid-length runs and a big effort on the weekend, with one or two easy days built in. In our 10-day phase, you'll get in an extra mid-long run and still have time to work different pacing and distances into your workouts, while also fielding an adequate amount of rest. For example, in Week 10 of our Advanced Training Program, we have you doing two steady-pace runs at 7 miles, an 8-mile run with a 3-mile pickup at marathon race pace, a 12-mile medium-long run, and a 20-mile-long run all in one 10-day cycle. You'll be running distances of 6, 7, 8, 12, and 20 miles, all at various speeds. That's how to best train for a marathon—you want to progressively increase the volume of your runs and at different paces, so that your body can adapt to running under more stress. Just remember that the harder you push it, the more time it needs to recover. That's why the 10-day phases in our Advanced Program include 1 day off and an average of 3 or 4 easy, recovery runs.

Picking Up the Different Paces

Before I get into each of the training programs, I want to familiarize you with some of the various pace workouts and key terms that will be vital to your training. These include easy, relaxed pace runs, long runs, mid-long runs, marathon-pace pickups, steady pace runs, and tempo pace runs. For intermediate and advanced runners, it's very important that you train at a variety of speeds and distances. I don't believe that speedwork on a track is of much use to beginning runners—more often than not, it only gets them injured—but you have to run at a faster tempo every once in a while, so that you're increasing your leg turnover and also applying more types of stress to your body. Eventually this will make your marathon pace feel a lot easier to you. Likewise, running more distances will also increase your cardio output and allow you to run with a greater, more efficient engine, if you will. The more time you spend on your feet, the easier the miles should come to you. It's also okay to be progressive in the sense that if you're feeling good, go ahead and run at a little faster than easy, recovery pace. Just remember that if you do have the urge to run faster, it becomes a harder workout and you'll need to follow it with an easy day or two.

Easy

Easy is just that—the effort is really low. It's very relaxed, meaning that you can have a conversation while you're running. If you can't, then your effort is too hard. This is the pace you want to use for both your long runs and mid-long runs, as well as your recovery runs (i.e., easy days). It should be approximately 50 to 90 seconds slower than marathon race pace. One of the hardest things for elite runners to do is to go for an easy, relaxed 8-mile run, yet it's one of the most valuable things they can do in their training. It gives their bodies a chance to recover from an extremely hard workout and helps flush out the excess lactic acid they've built up in their legs and repair all of the micro-tears to their muscles.

In all three programs, every long run is followed by an off day and then a relatively modest easy run, which gives your body nearly 2 days to recover. All the recent studies have borne out what Bowerman preached some 50 years ago: that if you train a body really hard and give it ample time to recover, it will come back stronger. The problem with the average runner today, however, is that he or she wants to train really hard all the time. Remember: Training has a cumulative effect, and if you're constantly running at marathon race pace, then you're more than likely to get hurt or sick and never make it to the starting line on race day.

Long Run

The long run is the longest and most important run during each phase of training. It is what every marathon training program is built around. Traditionally, most people think of it as 18 miles or more, but as you can see in Phase 1 of our Beginner's Program it can be as little as 6 miles. There really is no magic number attached to the long run, because everyone is different and what's most important is getting your body used to enduring, or on-your-feet time. Some beginners may never run 18 miles in their training, as that would require them to be on their feet for more than 3 hours, which is too long.

The general rule of thumb is that your long run should average out to roughly 25 percent of your weekly (or phase) mileage. This is why the length of the long run gradually increases from week to week, peaking at around 20 miles 3 weeks prior to your race. However, the total mileage should be of little concern to beginning marathoners, whose primary focus should be to spend a little more time on their feet each and every week. If they gradually increase the volume and time on their feet on their long runs to where they're used to enduring for 2½ to 3 hours, they should be able to meet the demands of running 26.2 miles.

Speed should never enter the equation on a long run, even for the advanced runner. *All* runs should be at approximately 65 to 70 percent of your maximum heart rate, or about 1 minute to 90 seconds slower than marathon race pace. (It might be

LONG-RUN PROTOCOL

The long run is one of the critical elements of any marathon training program. To accelerate the recovery process and make sure you rebound smoothly from these long, hard efforts, follow these six essential steps whenever possible.

1. Hydrate. The very first thing you should do is get your hands on some water and a sports drink loaded with sodium and electrolytes, especially if you're a heavy sweater.

2. Stretch. You can do this as you're hydrating. Make sure to stretch within 15 minutes after the completion of your run, while your muscles are still warm. (See chapter 7 for the best static, post-run stretches.)

3. Eat. You need protein to help facilitate the repair and rebuilding of muscle, and carbohydrates to replenish your depleted glycogen stores. There are plenty of energy bars out there that have both.

4. Control inflammation. Take some natural anti-inflammatory supplements such as fish oil, curcumin, or 1-TDC tablets within 30 to 60 minutes of your run. NSAIDs, such as Advil and Aleve, cause water retention and make you gain weight. If you find that the natural supplements are not doing the job, then take 2 to 4 pain relief tablets after the run (if not contraindicated by your doctor). The key is to not allow the inflammation to get out of control.

5. Break it down. If you can get a massage, do it. If not, a foam roller is a worthy substitute. It works just like a massage to break down soft tissue while increasing blood circulation to the muscle and tendon areas to speed healing.

> 6. Take a cold bath. Drop a couple of bags of ice in some cold tub water and chill out until the ice melts, or for about 10 minutes. This is the most effective way to control inflammation in your lower body after a long run.

closer to 50 seconds for the faster, well-trained athlete.) Don't use the long run as a barometer for the marathon, to see if you can sustain race pace for 20 miles. Many people make this mistake and pay dearly for it. It's simply too excessive and stressful on the body. Save this type of effort for marathon day. Provided that you gradually increase the volume and time on your feet, and incorporate a few faster tempo runs into your training from time to time, the speed part will come.

Mid-Long Run

The value to this workout is that it incorporates another distance run into your 10-day phase, and it's not as hard on the body as the long run. Like the long run, it should be performed at an easy, relaxed pace approximately a minute slower than marathon race pace. You'll still gain a substantial training effect by running slow and easy, because you'll be increasing your mileage and time on your feet. The trick to being a successful marathoner, whether you're a beginning, intermediate, or advanced runner, is to gradually get your body acclimated to running longer distances. Speed is strength in disguise, and much of your strength comes from running more—the more you run, the easier the action of running becomes.

Pickups

For intermediate and advanced runners looking to set a personal best or time-qualify, it's necessary to introduce a little speed and tempo at marathon race pace into your training. One way to accomplish this is to set out to run a desired distance at race pace in the middle of a medium-length run. These mid-run pickups, as Fleming likes to call them, are relatively short in duration (2 to 3 miles, sometimes more for the advanced runner), but they have the same effect as doing reps on a track, and they're safer. We have some 2- and 3-mile pickups at 7 and 8 miles in the Advanced Marathon Training Program and at 5 and 6 miles in the Intermediate Program. You should run at an easy, relaxed pace on either side of these pickups. Besides being a great confidence-booster, pickups help you establish a feel for your marathon race pace and differentiate it from other paces. More important, when you combine it with all the other forms of training in a 10-day phase, it mimics the fatigue you'll experience in the latter stages of the marathon when you're trying to maintain your race pace.

Steady

"Steady" is a word that Fleming uses to control the pace. It's very easy to confuse with the word *tempo*, but a tempo run has a very distinct goal and time in mind, such as running 5 miles at 9:20 pace (i.e., 10 to 15 seconds slower than marathon race pace). Steady means that you're going to go out and run the same pace over the entire distance. It's generally not as fast as tempo pace because it needs to be a pace that you can easily sustain the whole way. With a steady run, there is no mid-run pickup or sprint to the finish, or easy, slow miles; it's like setting your body on cruise control so that you can maintain a steady speed for the duration of your run.

Tempo

A tempo run imparts more stress on your body than a steady run. It's not quite marathon race pace, but it's certainly not easy, either. You're going to run at an effort of about 70 to 75 percent of your max heart rate, versus 65 to 70 percent for an easy run. Fleming believes that you'll see more improvement doing tempo runs than you will doing intervals, or speedwork. Intervals are very short in duration, whereas if you go out and run 6 or 7 miles at tempo pace, you're consistently stretching your effort out over a longer distance and amount of time. As you get more fit, your tempo should also improve and your pace will become easier and faster.

Beginner's Marathon Training Schedule

If you're a beginner or novice runner who's planning to run in your very first marathon, you may have run a half-marathon, 10K, or 15K before, and you likely have been running 20 to 25 miles per week for several months. This is very important—you need to have some type of strong cardio base before you begin training for a marathon. At minimum, you should be running 4 or 5 miles four to five times per week.

There are people who sign up to run a marathon in 6 months' time having never jogged more than 3 miles in their life. If this is you, I applaud you for pursuing your dreams and taking on such a worthy challenge; however, I would advise you to hold off for another year and follow a training regimen like the Run for Weight Loss and Life Training Plan in chapter 15, which will get you to a point where you can run 20 miles per week on a consistent, fairly easy basis. Get yourself fit and run in some local races to get a better sense for what kind of mileage and pacing you're capable of. Chances are that this will simply stoke your passion for next year's marathon even more. I don't want you to kill the fire; I just want you to build up your mileage so that you're better equipped to handle 4 months of hard, rigorous training.

The goal of the Beginner's Program is to get you running more, and at longer distances, so that you can learn how to comfortably run for 2½ to 3 hours. It's about building endurance and on-your-feet time, not speed, which is why you won't be doing any pickups or speedwork in this program. The fastest you'll be running is at a steady pace. I don't want you worrying about your marathon race pace at all, because the goal of any first-time marathoner should be to finish and enjoy the experience, not to try to qualify for Boston. Trust me, when you cross the finish line, you're going to feel a sense of overwhelming joy and accomplishment that no finish time can strip away. You can worry about your time on the next one.

The key to building that endurance is the long run. You'll see that we've attached distances to these long runs in the program, but that's only to give you a sense for the amount of effort and time that you'll be spending on your feet. There really is no magic number; you'll determine what pace comes easy and is relaxed and sustainable for you. What's more important is that you gradually build more and more time running on your feet, maxing out at 2½ to 3 hours in Phase 10. If you can run 18 miles in under 3 hours, then so be it, but I don't want you extending yourself beyond 3 hours. This is sufficient enough time to be on your feet, even if you think it's going to take you 5 hours to run the marathon. How are you going to be able to run the additional 2 hours come race day? That's easy: (1) You've got a bib on your chest—the adrenaline you get from the crowd and from being part of such a spectacle is worth 100 speed intervals; and (2) your aerobic endurance is 10 times what it was when you started training 4 months earlier.

We know that training is a struggle for beginners and that many get injured the very first go-around, which is why you have an off day on both sides of your long run and 4 days off in every phase except Phase 4. The idea behind having 4 off days is that we don't want you running more than 3 consecutive days. Yes, we want you on your feet more, but we do that by steadily increasing the mileage on your training runs. We feel that it's better for the beginning marathoner to rest too much rather than not enough. If you feel like 4 days off is too many, then by all means substitute an easy run for one or, better yet, do some light strength conditioning (see chapter 5) or cross-training (see chapter 6). Don't overexert yourself. Focus on running easy and relaxed, and increasing your volume, and you should have little trouble getting to the finish line.

Beginner's Marathon Training Schedule

	Day 1	Day 2	Day 3	Day 4	Day 5	
Phase 1	4mi easy	4mi easy	OFF	4mi easy	4mi easy	
Phase 2	4mi easy	4mi easy	OFF	7mi (long run)	OFF	
Phase 3	8mi (long run)	OFF	5mi easy	OFF	5mi easy	
Phase 4	5mi easy	OFF	5mi easy	OFF	10mi (long run)	
Phase 5	OFF	12mi (long run)	OFF	5mi easy	5mi easy	
Phase 6	5mi steady pace	OFF	6mi easy	6mi easy	OFF	
Phase 7	6mi easy	OFF	14mi (long run)	OFF	6mi easy	
Phase 8	6mi easy	OFF	7mi steady pace	OFF	8mi easy	
Phase 9	OFF	7mi easy	OFF	16mi (long run)	OFF	
Phase 10	7mi easy	OFF	6mi at steady pace	OFF	9mi easy	
Phase 11	OFF	5mi easy	5mi easy	OFF	12mi easy	
Phase 12	4mi easy	OFF	5mi easy	OFF	4mi easy	

Ledger

Easy: Conversational pace; relaxed; approximately 50 to 90 seconds slower than marathon pace.

Steady: A constant pace that is sustained over the entire duration of the run.

Long Run: Your longest run in each phase, roughly 25 percent of phase mileage; always run at easy pace.

Day 6	Day 7	Day 8	Day 9	Day 10	Total Mileage
OFF	6mi (long run)	OFF	4mi easy	OFF	**26**
4mi easy	5mi easy	OFF	5mi easy	OFF	**29**
5mi steady pace	OFF	5mi easy	5mi easy	OFF	**33**
OFF	5mi easy	5mi easy	5mi steady pace	OFF	**35**
5mi steady pace	OFF	6mi easy	6mi easy	OFF	**39**
13mi (long run)	OFF	6mi easy	OFF	6mi easy	**42**
5mi easy	6mi tempo pace	OFF	7mi easy	OFF	**44**
OFF	15mi (long run)	OFF	6mi easy	6mi easy	**48**
6mi easy	6mi easy	7mi at steady pace	OFF	8mi easy	**50**
6mi easy	OFF	18mi (long run)	OFF	6mi easy	**52**
OFF	5mi easy	5mi easy	5mi steady pace	OFF	**37**
3mi easy	OFF	OFF	**MARATHON**	OFF	**42.2**

30 MINUTES TO
A STRONGER, FASTER YOU

While it's tempting to relax and become a couch potato on your off days, your performance on race day will get a huge boost if you spend some additional time strength training. Just two 30-minute sessions per week will increase your lean muscle mass and, as a result, allow you to recruit more muscle fibers to help power your legs during those last few miles when they're completely out of gas. An additional benefit to these workouts is that they help strengthen the muscles and muscle-tendon junctions in your lower extremities, so you're less apt to get injured.

The following 30-minute workout is derived from the strength-building exercises in chapter 5. Walk briskly on the treadmill or outside for 5 to 10 minutes beforehand to make sure you're adequately warmed up. You could also ride a stationary bike or do the elliptical.

- Double- or single-leg calf raises (see page 61 for full description): Perform 2 sets of 15 reps.
- Standing leg kicks (page 63): Perform 100 kicks on each leg.
- Monster walks with resistance band (page 66): Perform 3 sets of 5 steps in each direction.
- Standing tree pose (page 70): Hold for 10 deep breaths in and out on both legs.
- Dumbbell hammer curls (page 76): Perform 2 sets of 15 reps using light weights (5 to 15 pounds).
- Regular or wall push-ups (pages 74 and 75): Perform 2 sets of 10 reps.

- Abdominal crunch (page 71): Hold for a count of 10 deep breaths in and out, 2 reps on each leg.
- Plank (page 69): Hold the pose two times for 45 seconds or more.

FOR WEEKEND WARRIORS

Most runners prefer to do their long runs on the weekends, usually on Sunday, because it's when they have the most free time. Since they typically don't have to go to work afterward, they can rest more efficiently. We understand this, which is why we've done our best to schedule as many long runs on a Saturday or Sunday as we possibly can in our 12-phase, 10-day-per-week plans. Unfortunately, Day 10 doesn't always fall on a Sunday, like Day 7 does in every 7-day plan, which presents some difficulties when trying to schedule a Sunday long run.

Every plan is amendable and can be changed to fit your schedule, provided you adhere to the basic hard-easy-easy rule and follow a long run with two easy recovery days and a hard effort with one or more easy days. Stay within those parameters, and you can accommodate your long runs on the weekend if necessary.

Intermediate Marathon Training Schedule

The intermediate runner is typically someone who has one or more marathons under his or her belt and is now more interested in achieving a personal best or breaking through some time barrier than in simply crossing the finish line. The latter is no longer good enough. This is your plan if you're looking to break 4 or 4½ hours or to best that 3:55 that your mom or dad did 25 years ago. Maybe you have experience running in a lot of races (10Ks, half-marathons), and you want to take a step up in class, or you trained for a marathon before and got injured. The Intermediate

Intermediate Marathon Training Schedule

	Day 1	Day 2	Day 3	Day 4	Day 5
Phase 1	4mi easy	4mi steady pace	4mi easy	6mi (mid-long run)	OFF
Phase 2	7mi (mid-long run)	OFF	4mi easy	10mi (long run)	OFF
Phase 3	5mi steady pace	4mi easy	11mi (long run)	OFF	4mi easy
Phase 4	5mi steady pace	12mi (long run)	OFF	5mi easy	5mi easy with 2mi pickup
Phase 5	13mi (long run)	OFF	5mi easy	5mi easy	8mi (mid-long run)
Phase 6	6mi easy	14mi (long run)	OFF	5mi easy	5mi easy
Phase 7	5mi easy	5mi easy	16mi (long run)	OFF	5mi easy
Phase 8	6mi easy with 2mi pickup	5mi steady pace	5mi easy	18mi (long run)	OFF
Phase 9	6mi easy	5mi easy	17mi (long run)	OFF	5mi easy
Phase 10	6mi easy	9mi (mid-long run)	OFF	6mi easy	6mi at marathon pace
Phase 11	OFF	5mi easy	5mi at marathon pace	4mi easy	10mi (mid-long run)
Phase 12	OFF	4mi easy	4mi tempo	OFF	4mi easy

Ledger

Easy: Conversational pace; relaxed; approximately 50 to 90 seconds slower than marathon pace.

Steady: A constant pace that is sustained over the entire duration of the run.

Pickup: A mid-run up-tempo workout in which you run 2 to 3 miles at marathon pace.

Tempo: Slightly faster and typically longer in duration than a steady pace; 70 to 75 percent of max heart rate.

Marathon Pace: Average pace per mile you aspire to run in the marathon (i.e., 7:30, 8:00, 8:30, etc.).

Long Run: Your longest run in each phase, roughly 25 percent of phase mileage; always run at easy pace.

Mid-Long Run: Additional moderate-length long run that helps build endurance and on-your-feet time.

ay 6	Day 7	Day 8	Day 9	Day 10	Total Mileage
ni easy	8mi (long run)	OFF	4mi easy	5mi steady pace	39
ni easy	4mi easy	5mi easy with 2mi pickup	4mi easy	5mi easy	44
ni eady pace	7mi (mid-long run)	OFF	5mi easy	5mi easy	46
ni (mid-long run)	OFF	6mi easy	5mi tempo pace	4mi easy	49
FF	6mi easy	5mi easy	5mi tempo pace	5mi easy	52
ni (mid-long run)	OFF	5mi easy	5mi easy	6mi easy with 2mi pickup	54
ni mpo pace	9mi (mid-long run)	OFF	5mi easy	6mi easy	56
ni easy	5mi steady pace	6mi easy	8mi (mid-long run)	OFF	58
ni easy with mi pickup	5mi easy	9 mi (mid-long run)	OFF	5mi easy	58
ni easy	20mi (long run)	OFF	5mi easy	5mi easy	62
FF	5mi easy	4mi easy	4mi easy	5mi easy	42
ni easy	OFF	3mi easy	**MARATHON**	OFF	45.2

Program is geared a little more toward speed and pace than the Beginner's Program, which is why we introduce the mid-long run, pickups, and more steady and tempo runs into this plan. Every phase has at least a tempo, steady, or pickup run in it, which helps you to turn your legs over more quickly and makes it easier to run at marathon race pace. The mid-run pickups simulate this race pace, which is why we put several in toward the end of your training, when you're running your peak mileage. At this point in your training, your legs should be feeling a little bit fatigued, just as they will come mile 20 on race day. It's very important that you're able to maintain race pace even when your legs aren't as well rested as they are at the beginning of your runs.

Just as in the Beginner's Program, building strength and aerobic endurance remains the biggest priority in the Intermediate Program. There are four planned long runs of at least 16 miles, plus several mid-long runs of 9 miles or more. Again, we've made sure to alternate hard and easy efforts so that each mid-long run and long run is followed by an off day and an easy recovery day. As is not the case in the Beginner's Program, however, your long run is not preceded by a day of rest. We've incorporated a short easy or tempo run to simulate a little more fatigue in the long run and to get your body best acclimated to what it'll experience on race day.

TRUST THE TAPER

If you've never tapered before, you should know that this time can be a little stressful, since the body is used to doing so much more. If you're starting to feel a little hypersensitive about everything in your training, then do some low-impact cross-training on the elliptical machine or StairMaster, or go for a nice, easy walk. Don't worry about losing your endurance, because you're still running—you're just not doing as much. Trust the work that you've put into your training and know that a well-rested, healthy body is a faster, more efficient body.

Advanced Marathon Training Schedule

If you're looking at our Advanced Program, then chances are that you're trying to meet the qualifying standard set for the Boston Marathon or some other race you've put high on your bucket list. Or maybe you're seeking to run a sub-3-hour marathon. It's likely that you've been running for years and have at least a half-dozen or more marathons under your belt. You compete in a lot of races and perhaps belong to a local running club.

For the 2014 Boston Marathon, the qualifying time for men ages 18 to 34 was 3 hours, 5 minutes, and for women of the same age group it was 3 hours, 35 minutes. These qualifying standards increase with age—for example, 3:15 for men ages 40 to 44, and 3:45 for women 40 to 44. Because of the time requirement, you're going to notice a steadier diet of up-tempo and race pace runs in the Advanced Program. As you can see, most of the mid-long runs are preceded by a steady run, and we've even introduced a few steady efforts prior to the long run, to boost the training effect of your long runs. In Phase 9, we've also introduced a 7-mile tempo run at marathon race pace. These hard tempo runs are a staple of the Kenyans' training programs, although they're more apt to run 22 miles instead of 7—albeit at a pace 5 to 10 seconds slower than race pace. These longer tempo runs will really test your cardiovascular fitness and help increase your VO_2 max so that a 7:20 race pace on marathon day feels a whole lot easier to sustain.

Still, your long run and mid-long run will continue to serve as the meat and potatoes of your training. By increasing your mileage and on-your-feet time and combining that with the variety of different paces you're training at, you should see a positive cumulative effect on race day. You should become more efficient at running faster at longer distances. Feel free to substitute some of your races for hard workouts, and resist the urge to get in an extra-long run during your taper (Phases 11 and 12). Many advanced runners have a hard time scaling back their training during this taper period, but you've got to give your body time to recover from training. So if you're going to keep running, then you must treat every day like it's a relaxed recovery day.

Advanced Marathon Training Schedule

	Day 1	Day 2	Day 3	Day 4	Day 5
Phase 1	6mi steady pace	6mi steady pace	6mi steady pace	8mi (mid-long run)	6mi easy
Phase 2	8mi (mid-long run)	5mi easy	6mi steady pace	12mi (long run)	OFF
Phase 3	7mi steady pace	6mi easy	14mi (long run)	OFF	7mi easy
Phase 4	7mi steady pace	14mi (long run)	OFF	6mi easy	7mi tempo pace
Phase 5	16mi (long run)	OFF	7mi easy	7mi steady pace	9mi (mid-long run)
Phase 6	7mi easy	16mi (long run)	OFF	6mi easy	7mi steady pace
Phase 7	6mi easy	7mi easy	18mi (long run)	OFF	7mi easy
Phase 8	6mi easy	7mi easy	7mi steady pace	20mi (long run)	OFF
Phase 9	7mi at marathon pace	6mi easy	20mi (long run)	OFF	6mi easy
Phase 10	7mi steady pace	12mi (mid-long run)	6mi easy	7mi steady pace	7mi at marathon pace
Phase 11	7mi easy	6mi easy	10mi (mid-long run)	6mi easy	OFF
Phase 12	7mi easy	6mi easy	6mi tempo	OFF	6mi easy

Ledger

Easy: Conversational pace; relaxed; approximately 50 to 90 seconds slower than marathon pace.

Steady: A constant pace that is sustained over the entire duration of the run.

Pickup: A mid-run up-tempo workout in which you run 2 to 3 miles at marathon pace.

Tempo: Slightly faster and typically longer in duration than a steady pace; 70 to 75 percent of max heart rate.

Marathon Pace: Average pace per mile you aspire to run in the marathon (e.g., 6:30, 7:00, 7:30, etc.).

Long Run: Your longest run in each phase, roughly 25 percent of phase mileage; always run at easy pace.

Mid-Long Run: Additional moderate-length long run that helps build endurance and on-your-feet time.

ay 6	Day 7	Day 8	Day 9	Day 10	Total Mileage
mi teady pace	12mi (long run)	OFF	7mi easy	7mi easy	63
mi easy	6mi steady pace	7mi easy	7mi easy with 2mi pickup	6mi easy	64
mi teady pace	8mi (mid-long run)	6mi easy	7mi easy with 2mi pickup	6mi easy	67
mi (mid-long run)	6mi easy	7mi easy	6mi easy with 2mi pickup	7mi easy	69
mi easy	6mi easy	7mi easy with 2mi pickup	6mi easy	7mi easy	71
0mi (mid-long run)	6mi easy	6mi easy	7mi easy with 2mi pickup	7mi tempo	70
mi steady pace	10mi (mid-long run)	6mi easy	6mi easy	8mi easy with 3mi pickup	75
mi easy	7mi steady pace	11mi (mid-long run)	7mi easy	7mi easy	79
mi easy	7mi steady pace	11 mi (mid-long run)	6mi easy	7mi easy	77
mi easy	20mi (long run)	OFF	6mi easy	7mi easy	78
mi at marathon pace	6mi easy	6mi easy	6mi steady pace	6mi easy	59
mi easy	OFF	3mi easy	**MARATHON**	OFF	53.2

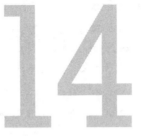

How to Run Your Best
Half-Marathon

AMERICANS ARE TAKING TO ROAD RACES MORE THAN EVER BEFORE, and their favorite distance might surprise you. It's not the marathon, the final track and field event of the Summer Olympic Games and the most celebrated distance; nor is it the 5K, which is popular because of its brevity (it's only 3.1 miles). No, for the past decade, more Americans have laced up their shoes to run the half-marathon than any other race.

According to Running USA's 2013 Half-Marathon Report, there were a record-high 1.85 million half-marathon finishers in 2012, a 14.9 percent increase from 2011. What's more, the number of finishers in the 13.1-mile event rose by 10 percent or more for the seventh consecutive year. Since 2000, the number of finishers of America's favorite race has more than quadrupled, from 482,000 to almost 2 million.

Women seem to have a particular fondness for the 21-kilometer distance, as they made up 60 percent (or 1.1 million) of all half-marathon finishers in 2012. In Running USA's 2013 National Runner Survey, 42.5 percent of all women surveyed chose it as their favorite race distance, and 80.5 percent said they'd be interested in running a half-marathon in 2013. Surprisingly, the marathon, with 41.1 percent, came in last (57.5 percent said they'd like to enter a 10K, and 57.1 percent a 5K).

Why so popular? For one, the M word—marathon. People today want to check the marathon off their bucket list, and it's much easier to run 13.1 miles than it is 26.2. Another reason is that many runners want to dip their feet in at 21 kilometers before they test their mettle at the actual marathon distance. While it's true that many first-time marathoners jump right in and never run so much as a 5-kilometer race before the big one, the half is a good barometer to see if you can handle the extra distance . . . and if you have the thirst for it. While the half doesn't require you to train for 16 to 18 weeks, like a full marathon does, it's not something you can afford to take lightly. You still need to train and put in the prep work—the three half-marathon plans that follow, for example, are 12 weeks long and have all the staples of a marathon training program, including long runs, tempo runs, and a taper.

Yet perhaps another explanation for the half's growing popularity is that it's a good "retirement" distance. By that, I mean that many veteran marathoners simply don't want to train for another full marathon, or put their bodies through one again. The half-marathon distance is much more manageable in terms of their goals, health, and time constraints, yet still provides a worthy challenge and an excuse to get out there almost every day to run. "The half-marathon is *half* as easy [as the marathon]," says Fleming, a 1:04:07 half-marathoner, explaining why he found the half distance appealing. "You can recover more quickly racing half-marathons, and it's not nearly as hard on the body."

Whatever your reasons are for running the half, here are three programs designed to get you to the finish line in the fastest, most efficient manner possible, whether you're a first-timer or you're trying to finish in under 1:30 for the first time.

Half-Marathon Beginner's Training Schedule

If you plan on running a full marathon one day, you really should consider running a half first, just to gain some valuable experience on what it's like to train for a longer-distance run. The beginner's program is designed for the first-time half-marathoner whose goal is to do just that—finish the race, and get a marathon-distance run under his or her belt. That's why you won't see any tempo runs or race pace pickups in this plan. It's not about speed; it's about learning how to endure and build more on-your-feet time.

In many ways, this plan is similar to the Beginner's Marathon Training Schedule in chapter 13, except that each phase, or training week, has been scaled back down to the normal 7 days. The idea is to increase your mileage slowly and get you to progressively run more and more. Do this consistently, and in 4 to 5 weeks' time, you'll start to feel yourself getting faster. All of your training efforts, including your long runs, should be run at an easy, relaxed pace, approximately a minute slower than your planned race day pace. If you're not sure what that is, then simply run at a conversational pace (i.e., being able to hold a conversation with a training partner as you run). There's no need to run any faster, because, once again, the goal is enduring, not speeding to the finish line. Introducing speed or tempo work is only likely to get you hurt, not ready for race day.

Half-Marathon Beginner's Training Schedule

	Day 1	Day 2	Day 3	Day 4	
Week 1	OFF	3mi easy	3mi easy	4mi easy	
Week 2	OFF	3mi easy	3mi easy	4mi easy	
Week 3	OFF	4mi easy	3mi easy	4mi easy	
Week 4	OFF	4mi easy	3mi easy	4mi easy	
Week 5	OFF	4mi easy	3mi easy	4mi easy	
Week 6	OFF	4mi easy	4mi easy	4mi easy	
Week 7	OFF	4mi easy	4mi easy	4mi easy	
Week 8	OFF	4mi easy	5mi easy	4mi easy	
Week 9	OFF	4mi easy	5mi easy	4mi easy	
Week 10	OFF	4mi easy	5mi easy	6mi easy	
Week 11	OFF	4mi easy	3mi easy	4mi easy	
Week 12	OFF	4mi easy	OFF	4mi easy	

Ledger

Easy: Conversational pace; relaxed; approximately 50 to 90 seconds slower than half-marathon pace.

Long Run: Your longest run of the week, roughly 25 percent of your weekly mileage; always run at easy pace.

Day 5	Day 6	Day 7	Total Mileage
OFF	3mi easy	5mi (long run)	18
OFF	3mi easy	5mi (long run)	18
OFF	5mi easy	6mi (long run)	22
OFF	6mi easy	7mi (long run)	24
OFF	6mi easy	7mi (long run)	24
OFF	7mi easy	8mi (long run)	27
OFF	7mi easy	8mi (long run)	27
OFF	7mi easy	9mi (long run)	29
OFF	7mi easy	9mi (long run)	29
OFF	7mi easy	10mi (long run)	32
OFF	5mi easy	8mi easy	24
OFF	3mi easy	**HALF-MARATHON**	24.1

Half-Marathon Intermediate Training Schedule

The intermediate runner has probably logged a few half-marathons before, and has a goal of running a personal best or breaking through some time barrier (e.g., finishing under 2 hours). These runners could also be scaling back from the longer marathon distance to give their body a break, or are simply motivated to try something new.

What's noticeably different about this plan in comparison to the Intermediate Marathon Training Schedule in chapter 13 is the presence of more faster-paced runs. Approximately 25 percent of your training runs will require you to run at race pace or faster than your normal relaxed, easy training pace (about 60 seconds slower than race pace). Outside of the first 2 weeks, there's a 5- or 6-mile tempo run each Tuesday and, in Weeks 3 through 10, a 6- or 7-mile run on Saturdays with a 2- to 3-mile pickup at half-marathon race pace or slightly faster. Remember: Half-marathon race pace is faster than marathon race pace, and tempo pace is closer to race pace than it is to training pace. Both require more effort than a simple training run, which places more stress on the body. This is important because your body needs to get stronger in order to meet the demands of running at a steady race pace for 13.1 miles. It has to get used to running at a faster tempo, and the best way to do that is to run progressively longer distances at a faster pace, closer to half-marathon pace, preferably in the middle to end of the program.

You'll still have your weekly long run, although it won't be as lengthy as those in the marathon plan. Your longest run will be 12 miles, in Week 10. As a result, you won't need as many easy recovery days as you do in the marathon plan. It's very important that you get your rest, however, which is why your weekends are preceded and followed by an off day. You have a 2- to 3-mile race pace pickup preceding your long run for 8 consecutive weeks. That's a tough weekend by any training plan's standards, and one that should get you more than ready for race day.

Half-Marathon Intermediate Training Schedule

	Day 1	Day 2	Day 3	Day 4	
Week 1	OFF	5mi easy	4mi easy	6mi easy	
Week 2	OFF	5mi easy	5mi easy	6mi easy	
Week 3	OFF	5mi tempo pace	5mi easy	6mi easy	
Week 4	OFF	5mi tempo pace	6mi easy	6mi easy	
Week 5	OFF	5mi tempo pace	6mi easy	7mi easy	
Week 6	OFF	5mi tempo pace	6mi easy	7mi easy	
Week 7	OFF	5mi tempo pace	6mi easy	7mi easy	
Week 8	OFF	5mi tempo pace	7mi easy	7mi easy	
Week 9	OFF	6mi tempo pace	7mi easy	7mi easy	
Week 10	OFF	6mi tempo pace	7mi easy	8mi easy	
Week 11	OFF	5mi tempo pace	6mi easy	7mi easy	
Week 12	OFF	5mi tempo pace	5mi easy	5mi easy	

Ledger

Easy: Conversational pace; relaxed; approximately 50 to 90 seconds slower than half-marathon pace.

Pickup: A mid-run up-tempo workout in which you run 2 to 3 miles at half-marathon pace.

Tempo: Slightly faster pace run at 70 to 75 percent of max heart rate.

Long Run: Your longest run of the week, roughly 25 percent of your weekly mileage; always run at easy pace.

Day 5	Day 6	Day 7	Total Mileage
OFF	5mi easy	6mi (long run)	26
OFF	6mi easy	7mi (long run)	29
OFF	6mi easy with 2mi pickup	7mi (long run)	29
OFF	6mi easy with 2mi pickup	8mi (long run)	31
OFF	6mi easy with 2mi pickup	8mi (long run)	32
OFF	6mi easy with 3mi pickup	9mi (long run)	33
OFF	7mi easy with 3mi pickup	9mi (long run)	34
OFF	7mi easy with 3mi pickup	10mi (long run)	36
OFF	7mi easy with 3mi pickup	11mi (long run)	38
OFF	7mi easy with 3mi pickup	12mi (long run)	40
OFF	6mi easy	8mi (long run)	32
OFF	3mi easy	**HALF-MARATHON**	28.1

Half-Marathon Advanced Training Schedule

If you fall into this group, you've probably run several half-marathons before, not to mention your fair share of marathons. And as with the marathon, you're not in this race to simply finish or coast through. You've got a goal of finishing in under 1:30 or maybe 1:20, and you want to push yourself to see how fast you can go. While not a 5K or a 10K, the half is still significantly shorter than the marathon; thus, you expect to run it faster and harder than you would a full marathon. That means your training is going to be anything but easy, even if it is 5 weeks shorter than the full-marathon training program.

The subtle differences in this plan versus the intermediate one are the progressively longer distances in the tempo and long runs (up to 8 and 15 miles, respectively) and the presence of an easy day prior to your long run. The easy recovery run acts as a buffer between your mid-run race pickups—the hardest effort of the week, according to Fleming—and your long runs, while still accomplishing the goal of making you run more. The tempo runs will get you to run at a variety of different distances (5 to 8 miles) and speeds—they should get slightly faster as you approach the middle and the tail end of your program. A 7-mile tempo run, in which you're conscious of maintaining the same pace throughout, can be a very hard, effective workout.

At any time, feel free to substitute a 5K or 10K race for one of your tempo workouts. If it happens to fall on your long run day, run the 10K and then 5 to 8 miles really slowly afterward, making sure to warm up sufficiently between the race and your easy, relaxed long run.

Half-Marathon Advanced Training Schedule

	Day 1	Day 2	Day 3	Day 4	
Week 1	OFF	5mi tempo pace	6mi easy	6mi easy	
Week 2	OFF	5mi tempo pace	6mi easy	6mi easy	
Week 3	OFF	6mi tempo pace	6mi easy	7mi easy	
Week 4	OFF	6mi tempo pace	6mi easy	7mi easy	
Week 5	OFF	7mi tempo pace	6mi easy	7mi easy	
Week 6	OFF	7mi tempo pace	6mi easy	7mi easy	
Week 7	OFF	7mi tempo pace	7mi easy	7mi easy	
Week 8	OFF	8mi tempo pace	7mi easy	7mi easy	
Week 9	OFF	8mi tempo pace	7mi easy	8mi easy	
Week 10	OFF	8mi tempo pace	7mi easy	8mi easy	
Week 11	OFF	7mi tempo pace	6mi easy	7mi easy	
Week 12	OFF	6mi tempo pace	6mi easy	5mi easy	

Ledger

Easy: Conversational pace; relaxed; approximately 50 to 90 seconds slower than half-marathon pace.

Pickup: A mid-run up-tempo workout in which you run 2 to 3 miles at half-marathon pace.

Tempo: Slightly faster pace run at 70 to 75 percent of max heart rate.

Long Run: Your longest run of the week, roughly 25 percent of your weekly mileage; always run at easy pace.

Day 5	Day 6	Day 7	Total Mileage
6mi easy with 2mi pickup	5mi easy	8mi (long run)	36
7mi easy with 2mi pickup	5mi easy	9mi (long run)	38
7mi easy with 2mi pickup	5mi easy	9mi (long run)	40
7mi easy with 2mi pickup	6mi easy	10mi (long run)	42
7mi easy with 3mi pickup	8mi easy	10mi (long run)	45
8mi easy with 2mi pickup	6mi easy	12mi (long run)	46
8mi easy with 3mi pickup	6mi easy	12mi (long run)	47
8mi easy with 3mi pickup	7mi easy	14mi (long run)	51
8mi easy with 3mi pickup	7mi easy	14mi (long run)	52
8mi easy with 3mi pickup	7mi easy	15mi (long run)	53
7mi easy with 2mi pickup	6mi easy	10mi (long run)	43
5mi easy	3mi easy	**HALF-MARATHON**	38.1

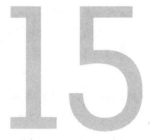

Run for Weight Loss and Life

ACCORDING TO THE CENTERS FOR DISEASE CONTROL AND PREVENTION, a staggering 68.8 percent of all American adults and one-third of all children are either overweight or obese. And because Americans are exercising less and less and consuming more sugar-sweetened beverages and foods, there's speculation that by the year 2030, more than half of the country's population will be obese.

Just what is obese? By definition, if your weight is significantly more than what is generally deemed healthy for your height, you're obese. More specifically, if you have a body mass index (BMI) of 30 or higher, you're considered obese; a BMI between 25 and 29.9 is considered overweight. You can calculate your BMI by dividing your weight in pounds by your height in inches squared and then multiplying this number by 703. Therefore, if you're 6 feet tall (72 inches) and your weight is 225 pounds, your BMI is 30.5 (225 ÷ 5,184 = .043 x 703 = 30.5). You would be considered obese.

The dangers of obesity have been well documented. Obesity is a contributing factor in five of the top ten leading causes of death—heart disease, cancer, stroke, diabetes, and kidney disease—among Americans. It can also lead to high blood pressure, sleep apnea, and depression. The American Medical Association recently classified obesity as a disease, and a big reason why this epidemic has become so serious is that Americans simply aren't exercising like they used to. According to a May 2012 report on obesity prevention from the Institute of Medicine, only 19 percent of Americans are getting the weekly recommended amount of physical activity they need—at least 150 minutes of moderate-intensity aerobic exercise per week, according to the American College of Sports Medicine. Too many children and adults are exercising their fingers (via the Internet, texting, and video games), but not their hearts.

Running is one of the best exercises you can do, not just for the body but for the mind as well. Sustained running has been shown to increase endorphin levels, and heightened endorphin levels enhance feelings of pleasure and help combat depression. It's also the ultimate cardiopulmonary/aerobic exercise and one of the most efficient ways to burn calories. When combined with the proper anti-inflammatory foods and supplements, running is a great way to keep yourself healthy and happy for a long time.

Statistics from Running USA's 2013 National Runner Survey bear this out. More than 17,000 female runners were surveyed, and their average BMI was 23.3, well below the overweight threshold. These women, on average, ran 3.9 days and 20.2 miles per week, and had been running for almost 10 years. The men in the survey of more than 30,000 core runners had an average weight of 174.4 pounds and a BMI of 24.7, again below the overweight threshold; they ran 4.1 days and 25.5 miles per week. Slightly more than 17 percent of the women and 15 percent of the men were motivated to start running because of weight concerns, and their primary motivation to continue running was to stay in shape (77.3 percent overall).

Running also has been shown to dramatically reduce insulin resistance, a condition in which a person's tissues have a lowered response to insulin, a powerful hormone made in the pancreas that helps to regulate the level of glucose (blood sugar) in the body. Insulin signals the body to store fat and glucose in cells while inhibiting the breakdown of fat. A diet that is high in sugars and trans fats increases inflammation and signals your body to create even more insulin. That's because the more insulin you have lingering in your bloodstream, the more resistant your body's insulin receptors become, and the more glucose and fat you store. This leads to weight gain and, in the most extreme conditions, diabetes.

The alarming rise in insulin resistance and obesity can be traced largely to the United States' ongoing embargo against Cuba, which dates back more than 50 years. Now most of our sugar is made from high-fructose corn syrup, the principal sweetener used in processed foods and beverages, and not natural cane sugar, which is too expensive. As a result, nearly every food product out there is processed with high-fructose corn syrup, including breads, cereals, condiments, and those soft drinks Americans love so much. In fact, in 2010, Americans consumed on average an astounding 60 pounds of high-fructose corn syrup per year, according to a Princeton University study. Researchers there found that rats with access to the sweetener gained significantly more weight than rats that received water sweetened with simple table sugar (the rats consumed the same number of calories). Long-term use of high-fructose corn syrup, researchers concluded, increases the overall risk of gaining abdominal fat and becoming obese.

You can decrease your insulin resistance and lower your risk of developing heart disease, strokes, and cancers by eating berries and other anti-inflammatory foods that increase your sensitivity to insulin. These foods include brightly colored fruits and vegetables, nuts, whole grains, and fish rich in vitamins, antioxidants, omega-3 essential fatty acids (EFAs), and fiber. Supplements such as fish oil (2,000 milligrams per day), curcumin (1,500 milligrams), vitamin D_3 (1,000 units), and wild blueberry capsules have also been shown to make you insulin-insensitive. Make sure to read the food labels and to avoid foods containing high-fructose corn syrup, preservatives (hydrogenated oil and trans fats), and saturated fats (animal fats, cooking oils), all of which increase the general level of inflammation in the body and raise your resistance to insulin. A good rule of thumb is to stay away from most packaged foods, bottled and canned beverages, and fast foods, which tend to be high in high-fructose corn syrup.

The other thing you can do, as mentioned, is to exercise more. Running is one of the best natural remedies for stimulating weight loss and combating obesity, especially when combined with a smart diet and the right supplements. The following Run for Weight Loss and Life Program is a relatively easy exercise plan designed to get you out there running and leading a more active, healthier lifestyle. The objective of the 18-week program is not to prepare you to run a marathon, but rather to get you fit enough so that you can run 16 to 20 miles per week. Consider this the first step in the process to running a marathon, if that should be one of your goals down the line. Before anyone should consider tackling a marathon, he or she must have a solid weekly base of about 20 miles per week.

There's growing evidence today that simply running as little as 6 miles per week can have tremendous health benefits, including increased insulin sensitivity and weight loss, stronger bones and muscles, a stronger heart and respiratory system, and a decreased risk for heart disease, high blood pressure, osteoporosis, and stroke. A ton of recent data also suggests that running helps keep the mind sharp and preserves brain function. Whether or not you're concerned about your weight, you simply can't ignore all the good things that running can do. For those of you who are not sure how to get started or simply need a little guidance and motivation, this is the right plan for you.

Run for Weight Loss and Life Program

The good news is there are no long runs or tempo runs in this program, and the only intervals alternate walking with running. Speed is not even a consideration. When you start running, you should do so at a relaxed, easy conversational pace. This is the pace our marathoners will use on their long runs and easy, recovery days. If you can't hold a conversation with someone as you're running, then you're probably going too fast. At first, you might struggle to talk and run at the same time, but as you get into the program, it should become very easy for you. Remember: The goal of this program is not to make you a 5K or 10K champion, but to get you running more regularly at whatever pace is comfortable to you. We're first going to get you walking every day, and then we'll slowly integrate running into the mix so that you're gradually building your endurance and tolerance for it.

The first week that you'll see any running is Week 3. You'll start with some quarter-mile intervals, in which you'll alternate walking and running every quarter mile up to a mile. This is also the first week that you'll have a rest day, which we'll designate as Thursday for the remainder of the program. The following week, you'll advance to half-mile walk/run intervals before running your first continuous mile (no intervals) in Week 5. The formula for the remainder of the program will be just as it is in Weeks 4 and 5, with the exception being that your intervals will be run/walk, not walk/run. Every 2 weeks, you'll increase your distance by a half mile, alternating between a week of intervals and a week of full-distance runs. Eventually, you'll get up to running 4 miles every other day in Week 17, or 16 miles per week. By Week 18, you should be able to run 16 to 20 miles per week, depending on your goals.

On your day off, it's a great idea to do some simple strength-training exercises, using your own body as resistance. This way, you can do them in the comfort of your own home. In fact, I recommend strength training at least twice per week for 30 minutes, or three times for 15 to 20 minutes. Calf raises, toe raises, single-leg kicks, mini-squats, wall push-ups, planks, and the standing tree pose are the best exercises for beginners (see chapter 5 for instructions on how to perform each exercise). You'll not only get a full-body workout, but you'll also strengthen those important weight-bearing muscles, bones, and tendons in your lower limbs so that you'll be better able to withstand the pounding that your body can take when running.

Run for Weight Loss and Life Training Schedule

	Day 1	Day 2	Day 3	Day 4	
Week 1	walk 20 minutes	walk 20 minutes	walk 20 minutes	walk 20 minutes	
Week 2	walk 30 minutes	walk 30 minutes	walk 30 minutes	walk 30 minutes	
Week 3	1mi (¼mi walk/run intervals)	walk 30 minutes	1mi (¼mi walk/run intervals)	REST	
Week 4	1mi (½mi walk/run intervals)	walk 30 minutes	1mi (½mi walk/run intervals)	REST	
Week 5	1mi run	walk 30 minutes	1mi run	REST	
Week 6	1½mi (½mi walk/run intervals)	walk 30 minutes	1½mi (½mi walk/run intervals)	REST	
Week 7	1½mi run	walk 30 minutes	1½mi run	REST	
Week 8	2mi (½mi walk/run intervals)	walk 30 minutes	2mi (½mi walk/run intervals)	REST	
Week 9	2mi run	walk 30 minutes	2mi run	REST	
Week 10	2½mi (½mi walk/run intervals)	walk 30 minutes	2½mi (½mi walk/run intervals)	REST	
Week 11	2½mi run	walk 30 minutes	2½mi run	REST	
Week 12	3mi (½mi walk/run intervals)	walk 30 minutes	3mi (½mi walk/run intervals)	REST	
Week 13	3mi run	walk 30 minutes	3mi run	REST	
Week 14	3½mi (½mi walk/run intervals)	walk 30 minutes	3½mi (½mi walk/run intervals)	REST	
Week 15	3½mi run	walk 30 minutes	3½mi run	REST	
Week 16	4mi (½mi walk/run intervals)	walk 30 minutes	4mi (½mi walk/run intervals)	REST	
Week 17	4mi run	walk 30 minutes	4mi run	REST	
Week 18	4–5mi run	walk 30 minutes	4–5mi run	REST	

Day 5	Day 6	Day 7	Total Mileage
walk 20 minutes	walk 20 minutes	walk 20 minutes	walk only
walk 30 minutes	walk 30 minutes	walk 30 minutes	walk only
1mi (¼mi walk/run intervals)	walk 30 minutes	1mi (¼mi walk/run intervals)	4mi walk/run
1mi (½mi walk/run intervals)	walk 30 minutes	1mi (½mi walk/run intervals)	4mi walk/run
1mi run	walk 30 minutes	1mi run	4mi run
1½mi (½mi walk/run intervals)	walk 30 minutes	1½mi (½mi walk/run intervals)	6mi walk/run
1½mi run	walk 30 minutes	1½mi run	6mi run
2mi (½mi walk/run intervals)	walk 30 minutes	2mi (½mi walk/run intervals)	8mi walk/run
2mi run	walk 30 minutes	2mi run	8mi run
2½mi (½mi walk/run intervals)	walk 30 minutes	2½mi (½mi walk/run intervals)	10mi walk/run
2½mi run	walk 30 minutes	2½mi run	10mi run
3mi (½mi walk/run intervals)	walk 30 minutes	3mi (½mi walk/run intervals)	12mi walk/run
3mi run	walk 30 minutes	3mi run	12mi run
3½mi (½mi walk/run intervals)	walk 30 minutes	3½mi (½mi walk/run intervals)	14mi walk/run
3½mi run	walk 30 minutes	3½mi run	14mi run
4mi (½mi walk/run intervals)	walk 30 minutes	4mi (½mi walk/run intervals)	16mi walk/run
4mi run	walk 30 minutes	4mi run	16mi run
4–5mi run	walk 30 minutes	4–5mi run	16–20mi run

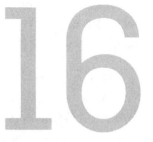

Race Day Strategies

THE BIG DAY HAS ARRIVED. YOU'RE ON THE BUS TRAVELING TO THE start of the marathon, and you're using this final bit of quiet time to get yourself fueled and mentally ready for the challenge that lies ahead. Now is not the time to be second-guessing your training (Did I train hard enough?) or the outfit you picked out several months earlier. Nor is it the time to be plotting a new strategy for the race in terms of pacing. You should try to relax and embrace the moment because the hard part—the months of training—is behind you. The marathon is relatively easy compared with all the months of training you put in. Certainly you can get through another 26.2 miles, especially with all that extra adrenaline you'll be carrying, not to mention the energy boost you'll get from the crowds along the way.

Here are some strategies for race day that should help you to accomplish your goal, whether it's to finish or to run a personal best:

Know That You've Done All the Work You Possibly Could Have Done

Running coach Tom Fleming is notorious for his work ethic. He is famous for saying, "Somewhere in the world, someone is training when you're not, and when you race him, he will win." While not the most talented or physically gifted runner (being taller and bigger than most), he was able to rise above his build and become one of the elite marathoners in the world because he trained harder than anybody else. You don't have to run nearly as much as he did, but if you're consistent in your training, and you progressively increase your mileage from week to week, you will improve, whether you're a 5- or a 2½-hour marathoner.

"I hear, 'Well, I felt great for 20 miles,' so many times," Fleming says. "Then it's all downhill from there. They're dead tired for the last 10K because they're undertrained. In the marathon, once you start going downhill, it's a steep hill to climb." But if you've stuck to the training plans in this book, you'll be thoroughly conditioned and can rest easy in the knowledge that you're as prepared for this race as you could possibly be.

Get a Road Map

You're probably not going to get the chance to preview the marathon course before you run it—unless, of course, you've competed in the race before. You can't run the streets of New York, London, or Boston prior to the event, unless you've got a special police escort at 4 in the morning. The good news is that most race websites have a map of the course, so you can see where it is you'll be running and what you can expect over the last few difficult miles of the course. Some sites also have a virtual map of the course so that you can identify where the steepest hills are during the race. At the New York City Marathon Health and Fitness Expo, you can even view all 26.2 miles of the course in real time, in a matter of just minutes.

"To know where you are when you race is a huge advantage, I think," Fleming says. "Some people run races and have no idea where they are. For example, a lot of runners don't know that you exit Central Park onto Central Park South at mile 25 [during the New York City Marathon]. It helps to know how the race is going to finish, whether you're turning left or right or going straight."

Imagine your surprise if you didn't know Heartbreak Hill was coming shortly after mile 20 in the Boston Marathon, or if you were oblivious to the long, gradual incline on the Queensboro/59th Street Bridge at mile 16 of the New York City Marathon. You don't want to be caught off guard, because that can leave you very flustered and distraught. It's also very helpful to know the topography of the course well in advance of the race, so that you can design your training to simulate these conditions. If you're running New York for the first time, you need to incorporate hills into your training because there are a lot of them on the course, especially over the last 10 miles. As for Boston, you want to learn how to run downhill as fast as you run uphill, says Fleming, and also include more up-tempo runs in your training, since the course is faster than the one in New York.

Don't Try Anything New on Race Day

The marathon is not the time to be trying out a new-brand pair of running shoes, a new sports drink or energy bar, or anything new, for that matter. A lot of runners buy race-specific shirts and clothes the week of the race and then wear them for the very first time on race day, then wonder why they're chafing 2 hours into the run. Don't wear anything without first giving it a test drive or two before race day. That includes everything from your socks to what sunscreen you're applying on your neck and face. The same goes for food and beverages as well. You don't want to try sushi for the first time the night before the marathon, or eat peanut butter and jelly right before the race when you've never done so before.

Everything you eat, drink, wear, and use on race day should already have been tested out during long runs in your training months, which not only serve to build endurance and strength but also double as dress rehearsals for the marathon. Wear exactly what you plan to on race day, and eat the same meal as well, both the night before and the morning of your last few long runs. If your plan is to alternate between water and Gatorade every mile or two during the marathon and to consume a packet of PowerGel or GU once every 45 minutes, then do that as well.

Use your final long run as a dry run for marathon day, from the time you wake up to the actual start time of the race. If, for example, you're running the New York City Marathon and you need to be up at 4:30 a.m. to catch the 5:45 bus to the start in Staten Island, then get up at 4:30, eat, warm up, and then go for your run at 10, 10:20, or whatever your scheduled start time is. Practice what it is you're going to do on race day, so that you're acclimated to the time and the process and there are no surprises for you on that day.

With regard to the shoes: If you insist, the new synthetic materials today make it possible to run in a new pair on race day, but only if it's the same make and model you've been running in for the past several months. Replace the insert with your old one and you should be good to go, says Fleming. However, if it's an entirely new brand or model, then you want to get several runs in first to break them in. You should complete at least one long run and log as many as 50 to 100 miles in them, to be safe.

Prepare for Any Type of Weather

At the 2012 Boston Marathon, unseasonably warm temperatures soared into the 80s, sending more than 100 runners to the hospital and causing another 4,300 registered runners to sit out the race entirely. Many of these runners trained during the cold winter months in the Northeast and were simply no match for the heat. They were expecting cool, comfortable running temperatures in the 40s or 50s, not sauna-like conditions.

In extremely hot weather, it's vital that you stay hydrated and consume more electrolytes than you normally would during a run. Don't drink only water, because it doesn't have the electrolytes your body needs. Good sources of electrolytes include sports drinks such as Gatorade and Powerade, and energy gels and chews. Before the race, take some salt tablets or supplements with water, or eat a snack high in sodium, like salted pretzels

Wear light-colored, breathable materials that wick sweat away from your skin, and make sure to wear a visor or a sweat-wicking race cap to keep the sun off much of your face. About half of your body's heat is dissipated through your head, so if you can, wear a visor to allow your head to breathe. You don't want a hat that's made of heavy materials, which will get bathed in sweat very quickly.

If you're running in a late spring, summer, or early fall marathon, when temperatures can be high, or in a typically warm destination such as Florida or Arizona, make sure you expose yourself to the heat in your training. Don't run inside on a treadmill every time the thermometer hits 80 or above. The more acclimated your body is to the heat, the less salt you excrete through your sweat, and the less chance you have of suffering from electrolyte depletion. In essence, your body has an easier time coping with the heat.

The same thing goes for the cold weather—get yourself acclimated to running in cooler conditions, if you can, so you're not caught off guard if the temperature is in the low 30s come race day. If it's unseasonably cold, make sure you stay hydrated, because it's easy to ignore those water stations when you're not sweating as much and are not as thirsty. Drink more water than Gatorade, because your body doesn't lose as much salt in cool, dry conditions. In cold weather, you lose most of your heat through your head, so it's important to keep your head covered. It's also critical to keep the outer extremities (fingers, hands, feet, toes, ears) warm, since they receive less blood flow than many other parts of your body. In many of the bigger events, such as New York, you're waiting around at the start for several hours, so make sure you bring along an old sweatshirt, a pair of sweatpants, gloves, a hat, and any other disposable items that will keep you warm. You don't want your body getting cold and stiff prior to the start of the race, and you also don't want to be doing jumping jacks for 2 hours to keep yourself warm, either. Better to come over-prepared than to freeze your duff off. Once you get going and warm up, you can peel these extra layers off and discard them in clothing donation bins by the starting line.

Ease into It

At the 2011 New York City Marathon, the average split difference between the first and second halves of the race for the entire field was plus 52 minutes, whereas it was a negative 2 minutes for the winner, Geoffrey Mutai of Kenya. Only 1.6 percent of the entire field negative split, like Mutai, who set a course record in the process (2:05:06). Mutai's slowest 5-kilometer split in 2011 was the first 5K, at 15:34. His three fastest splits were 14:41 (30K), 14:31 (35K), and 14:26 (40K). His last official 5K split was more than a minute faster than his first. He was able to negative split over the second half because he started out slow and relaxed, by his standards; he didn't jump out of the gate running as if he were being chased by a herd of wild buffalo.

As for the rest of the field, many of the runners did just the opposite and started too fast, running out of gas over the last 13.1 miles, as evidenced by the nearly 1-hour time difference between the first 21 kilometers and the second.

"Know that the marathon is an endurance race," Fleming says. "It runs 42 kilometers, which sounds even more intimidating than 26.2 miles. It's supposed to be hard. Knowing that will keep you calm and more relaxed at the beginning. If you go out faster than you did on your hardest training runs, you're going to die in the end."

That's hard to do at the Boston Marathon, where the first 6 or 7 miles are relatively flat or downhill. In fact, the first mile drops 130 feet! Even New York goads you into starting too fast. After the first mile on the Verrazano-Narrows Bridge, which is the steepest on the course, mile 2 is all downhill as you charge into the Bay Ridge section of Brooklyn. John Honerkamp, New York Road Runners' manager of runner products and services, had to pace American short-track speed skater Apolo Ohno in the 2011 marathon. It was Ohno's very first full marathon, and his goal was to break 3:40. (Ohno's sponsor, Subway, said it would donate $26,200 to the Special Olympics if he finished in under 4 hours.) After running a very modest 9:03 for the first mile, they ran the second mile in 7:12, evidence of how difficult it is to apply the brakes on this hill, especially after the steep incline and congestion that bottles you up in mile 1.

Honerkamp, an eight-time All–Big East runner at St. John's University in the mid-1990s and a virtual running coach for New York Road Runners' online training programs, tries to get his students to start out 20 to 30 seconds slower than marathon race pace, then bring the pace gradually down until they're eventually running even with or faster than marathon pace for the last 10 kilometers.

"If the course is flat, I tell people they should aim to run negative splits," says Honerkamp, a semifinalist in the 800 meters at the 1996 U.S. Olympic Trials. "It's hard to do that in New York because it's so hilly, but it helps people not to go out too fast."

Ohno, despite being a rookie to the marathon, wanted to go much faster than the 3:40 pace (8:23 per mile) he set out to run at the start. Being the speed skater he is, Ohno—the most decorated American Winter Olympic athlete of all time, with eight medals—often tried to turn the marathon into a speed track event. Honerkamp reined Ohno in by telling him that his splits were much faster than they actually were. It was the only way to get him to run even or negative splits in the end.

"He'd ask me what pace we were running, and I'd say, '7:30,'" Honerkamp says, noting that Ohno did not have a watch. "Instead, we were running 8:15, 8:12, 8:08. We ended up running a 7:49 average [per mile] and 3:25 with a 4-minute negative split. It's tough to negative split, because you have to be very patient, but I kind of forced him to do it." Thanks to Honerkamp, Ohno was able to hold his pace and beat his target, so Subway donated $26,200—$1,000 per mile run—to the Special Olympics.

Fleming believes that most runners should strive to run an even pace from start to finish, staying within 10 seconds on either side of their goal pace. It's also critical, he says, to have a plan in place and to know where it is you want to be, at various splits (10K, 13.1 miles, 20 miles) throughout the race.

"It's important to see your split times, to know that you're on pace for the first 20 miles," he says. "That can provide a huge, huge lift, knowing you just have to maintain the same pace for 6 more miles."

10 Additional Tips for Marathon Day

Here are a few other things you need to consider on race day and in the days leading up to the marathon:

1. Manage the Clock: Just as your body needs time to acclimate itself to the heat and cold, it needs time to adjust to travel across several time zones. For every hour difference there is between your home (i.e., where you trained) and the location of the race, you need to arrive a day earlier. For example, if you're running Boston and you live in London year-round (a 5-hour time difference), you need to arrive in New England at least 5 days prior to the race. That will give your body enough time to adjust to the time change and get back into a normal rhythm.

2. Rest Early: Make sure to get a good night's sleep (at least 8 hours) two nights before the marathon, because on the evening of the race, you'll be lucky to get more than a few hours' sleep. If you're running New York, you may need to get up as early as 4:30 a.m. to catch a bus or other transportation to the start of the race. Factor that in along with your nerves and concerns about what you're going to eat, going to the bathroom, etc., and it's easy to see why sleep is hard to come by.

3. Pack the Night Before: Lay out your clothes and essentials the night before the race, including your race bib, ID, cellphone, energy gels, etc., so you're not scrambling to put it all together in the early hours of the morning. If you're rushing out the door, you're liable to forget something. I'd recommend you pack your own roll of toilet paper, too, because you don't want to find yourself in the Porta-Potty empty-handed if it's run out. Bill Rodgers was notorious for sticking a wad of toilet paper in his sock, and Fleming used to put it in his waistband. "The more stuff you can do to be prepared for what you're not ready for, the better off you are," Fleming says.

4. Drink Up: Start hydrating in the days leading up the race, particularly the day before the marathon. Fleming would drink water to the point where he was sick of it. The better hydrated you are, the less likely you are to suffer from fatigue, cramping, or heat-related illnesses during the race. Check the color of your urine each time you go to the bathroom—if it's pale and looks like lemonade, you're sufficiently hydrated; if it's darker in color and resembles apple juice, you're not getting enough fluids.

5. Kick Your Feet Up: So many out-of-towners come to a place like Boston or New York and can't resist the urge to play tourist the day before the marathon. Save the museums and the shopping for a few days after the race, or the next time you're in town. If you're walking around all day, you're going to be toast on race day. Relax and stay off your feet as much as possible. Go to see a Broadway show or a movie or take in a ballgame.

6. Warm Your Legs Up: Thirty minutes prior to the start of the 1981 Los Angeles Marathon, Fleming jogged the 2 miles from his hotel to the start of the race near the Hollywood Bowl, race singlet in hand. He had just enough time to go to the bathroom and then off he went, running one of the fastest races (2:13:14) of his career. Most elite runners will jog an easy 1½ or 2 miles as a warm-up before the marathon, just not so close to the start of the race. You should also try to get in some kind of warm-up about 30 minutes to an hour before the race. That can be difficult to do in New York and other bigger marathons, where there's so little room to warm up. But if space is limited, try running in place or down the block and back several times, or do some jumping jacks or leg swings—nothing too strenuous that will wear you down.

7. Crest the Hills: When you encounter a steep climb such as Heartbreak Hill in Boston or the Queensboro/59th Street Bridge in New York, don't panic. And certainly don't attack it. Settle into an easy, relaxed pace and stay there. Maintain the same pace over the crest of the hill and down onto the downhill side. Many runners forget that there's another side and they go on vacation (i.e., give themselves a short rest) at the top of the hill. Instead, keep your momentum going and use it to propel you down the hill.

8. Split Up the Pie: When running a marathon, the whole is a lot scarier than the sum of its parts. That's why whether you're running the 26.2 miles for the very first time or the twenty-fifth, it helps to break up the distance into smaller chunks. Fleming used to view the marathon in three parts: halfway (13.1 miles), 20 miles, and the last 6.2 miles (10K). That's a good way to divide it up, because most runners are just trying to hang on those last 10 kilometers. If you can stay on your feet for 20 miles or maintain a reasonably even pace till then, you'll know that the ultimate goal is well within reach. Think about it—once you hit 20 miles, or about the same length as your longest long run, you've just got one 10K race left. With all the training you've done over the past 4 months, you could do that 10K in your sleep!

9. Find Your Happy Place: At some point during the marathon, you're going to feel pain, discomfort, and fatigue, especially during the last 10 kilometers. You'll probably start to doubt yourself as well, whether it be finishing the race or meeting your time goal. When you hit this low point, you have to dig down deeper and find a way to keep moving. Fleming used to convince himself that the last 6 miles of the marathon, no matter where he raced, was the small 6-mile training loop he did back home in New Jersey. He could run those 6 miles blindfolded if he had to, and if he pictured himself running on this training loop for the 1,000th time, it gave him the confidence boost he needed to finish the last 10 kilometers strong. Much of the marathon is mental, and sometimes you have to play little games with yourself to keep your mind off the big picture and the exhaustion you may be feeling. Use whatever mental tricks you've got.

10. Finish with Your Head Held High: First-time half or full marathoners should remove the word *just* or *simply* before the word *finish*, because to imply that running 13.1 or 26.2 miles is merely ordinary is not doing the feat justice. Any way you slice it, finishing a distance event is an extraordinary achievement, and enduring for 42 kilometers is something you'll look back on for the rest of your life with a tremendous sense of accomplishment and pride.

Acknowledgments

First off, I would like to thank my coauthor, Dave Allen, for encouraging me and being the force behind this book. Ever since he and I finished work on *Golf Rx* (Gotham Books, 2007), he's been nudging me to do a running book. It took some convincing on his part, but I'm glad we took this journey together.

Much gratitude to Tom Fleming for putting together the best training plans and lending his coaching eye to this project. If my daughter and son one day become competitive long-distance runners, I want Tom coaching them.

Many thanks to my team at Avery Publishing—Megan Newman, Gigi Campo, and Bill Shinker—for believing in my vision, and to Fred Vuich, for making the many exercises you see in this book come to life with his photography. Special thanks also to our models, Ariel Kiley and John Honerkamp, for lending us their legs and talents.

I would also like to thank professors Matthew Moran, PhD, and Shawn Williams, DC, PhD, as well as my many colleagues here at the Hospital for Special Surgery in New York, including doctors Joseph Feinberg, Howard Hillstrom, James Kinderknecht, Robert Marx, Struan Coleman, and Rock Positano, and sports nutritionist Heidi Skolnik, for their contributions to the book. A big thank you as well to Dr. Michael Fredericson of Stanford University and Patricia Ladis, PT, of KIMA Center for Physiotherapy and Wellness for her help with the dynamic stretches in chapter 7.

Finally, much thanks to Mary Darling and Dan Murphy for their help with this project, and my wife, Dilshaad, for turning running into our family sport.

Index